TEN STEPS to Control Diabetes

Mark E. Meijer, M.D.

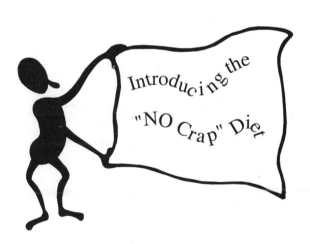

Introducing the "NO Crap" Diet

TEN STEPS to Control Diabetes

MeMend Books
toll-free 877-MeMend8

www.diabetesbook.info

ISBN: 0-9761572-0-9

Printed and bound in the United States of America

First Printing September 2004

To my children,

Erik and Jeana

TABLE OF CONTENTS

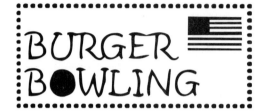

"AAAAGH!"

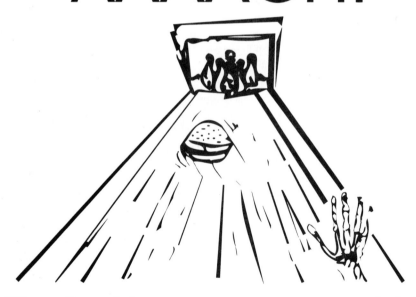

Whose funeral do you want to go to: yours or theirs?

1. Understand How to Succeed

Rome was not built overnight. Neither were you. Rome didn't fall apart overnight. Neither did you. Fixing your problems will take time too. If you keep doing the same things, you will keep getting the same results. If there is no need to change, why bother? If there is a need to change, why stop? The treatment of diabetes will become a lifestyle change; but it's not a lifestyle change unless it's done everyday.

If we do fail to "mend our ways," it is because lifestyle changes are hard to do. If needed transformation was easy, you probably would have done it a long time ago. Maintaining change can be even harder.

Let's face it: we hate to have to change and we can't change about how we feel about change. However, how we think about change can change . . . Huh?

Let's just keep this short and less painful.

Just read 1-3 chapters per day. Use a highlighter to highlight points that hit home with you. The next day reread some of this important (highlighted) points before putting the book away. Establish this ritual as a daily routine. If you read too much in one day, you won't remember enough of the extra reading to use it and it will only become a waste of your time. Overdoing anything can become an excuse to do nothing the following day. If it takes too long to do something one day, you won't have time to do it everyday and then it's not a lifestyle change.

Time yourself to determine how much you can read. Perhaps 10-15 minutes per day? Any extra time you do use reading cannot be saved for another day. Then try to keep in mind some of today's reading to see how you can fine-tune your health that day. Read, think, and then do something. *TEN STEPS To Control Diabetes* will give you goals that cannot be done in just one day. This is one reason why short chapters precede each step of "Ten Steps."

A little knowledge can help you if you do something better that day. If any step or goal seems too big, make it smaller. Bigger isn't always better. Faster isn't always better. Remember the story about the turtle and the rabbit that raced? Slower, small and smarter, the turtle won.

Anyone can do better. Times change from time to time; fools don't. It is time to make changes. Why not today? This doesn't have to take any longer than a trip to the bathroom.

If the need is there, wouldn't you go to the bathroom? If you don't have time to go to the bathroom, then you don't have time to stay alive (or read this book). If you can't make time to go to the bathroom, bigger problems than those that you have now will form and I can't help you. No one can. There are are things in life you must do, and only you can do it.

If you need to go now, GO! It can be that simple.

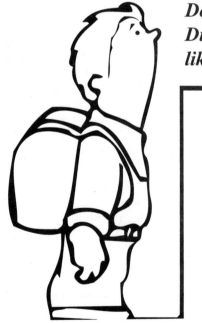

Does controlling Diabetes look like this?????

STEP ONE

TRY SMALLER STEPS!

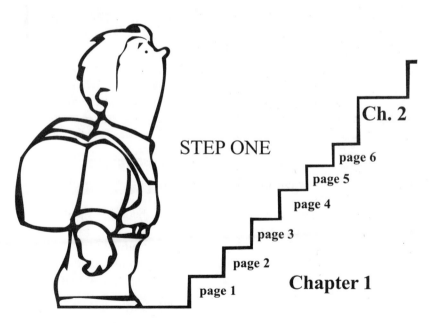

STEP ONE

Ch. 2

page 6

page 5

page 4

page 3

page 2

page 1

Chapter 1

2. How to Use This Book

The problems of learning about diabetes are similar to learning how to drive. Your first question might be, where should I begin? Your ultimate goal is to go somewhere, otherwise, why learn to drive? But when people are learning to drive for the first time, they are not too sure of themselves. It doesn't take long before there are a lot more questions to ask... like... how does one start the motor?

Before you actually drive, it is good to know two things: what is a car and what are the rules for the highway. For a diabetic, that means you need to know what diabetes is and what the rules are to control it.

The state you live in will provide you with a book on traffic rules. These rules are not negotiable. Neither are the rules for good diabetic control that this book provides.

You can learn about a car by reading the owner's manual. But you really have to sit at the controls before all that information starts to become understandable. A diabetic patient is the "controls" for diabetes. But where is the owners's manual for diabetes? You are reading it!

This book is your owner's manual and your rule book. I teach you what diabetes is. Knowing this should make it easier for you to control your diabetes. But you are not going to learn everything in one day, so don't try. Read new chapters when you are ready. Don't just read; understand and learn.

Most people drive their car every day. Even the worst drivers can get pretty good with daily practice. Repetition aids retention. Be patient, but persevere. Practice makes perfect.

It's not only a book you should read, it's a book you should reread! Repetition aids retention, that's how you learn.

Every chapter is small and a little story by itself. The first few chapters simply tell you what diabetes is. When you become familiar with the controls, we then introduce you to some of the rules you need to follow. If you don't like the rules, we try to explain to you, in simple terms, what the

Step 1

penalties are if you ignore the rules. You will learn where you can go. But getting there, ultimately, becomes your responsibility.

Many diabetics struggle because they cannot see what their goals are. All the "rules" and goals in this book are easy to understand. For many people, following them is what may be hard to do. In other words, it's not hard to see where you need to go, rather, it can be hard going there. I can't always make things easy to do, but I sure can make them easier to see.

Once you become familiar with the chapters you are studying and working on, you can move on to the next few. Some chapters require your attention for the rest of your life, if you want to do well. As with driving, negligence leads to problems. Use it or lose it. Practice makes perfect.

One of the hardest goals is losing weight, especially if you have been overweight (obese, fat, etc.) for a long time. You are not alone if you have this problem. If it was easy to lose weight, there wouldn't be so many fat people. More than half the country is overweight. Obesity in America is "normal."

If you have been obese for a long time, we discourage you from making weight loss your first or only goal. On the other hand, diet is an unavoidable four letter word that has to be addressed. And if you are an overweight diabetic, you will need to at least control weight, if not lose weight.

There is a right and a wrong way to lose weight. I will show you both and let you choose. The right way is for good health (to live), but it is not the easiest way. If staying alive is not important, losing weight is easy. Dead people lose weight.

Some diabetics struggle with other issues, even though for many obesity is always the biggest problem. Some need to quit smoking. Others can't afford the medicine. Some can't remember to take their medicine. If you can't read well, finding someone who will read this book to you might be the problem. Whatever it is, we all find things that are hard for us to do, but easy for someone else to do.

So you're not perfect. Neither am I.

STEP 1

But every diabetic must decide whether or not he or she wants to stay alive. If you are unsure, let your doctor know. I assume you do want to live and everything in this book assumes you have this goal in mind. So my primary concern should be your ultimate goal, which is a simple question to ask.: Do you want to live?

Your response should be; "YES, I want to live."

Most people are not going to do something difficult or painful without knowing why it has to be done. If I ask you to jump out of a three story building, I am sure you will say NO (if you want to live). But if I can convince you the building is on fire and jumping is your only means of escape, you might reconsider. In other words, it is helpful to know why you have to jump before you jump. To make things easier, I will try to soften the landing (e.g., add some pillows).

But ultimately, your choices are very simple. If you want to live, eat like it. None of the basic dietary goals, that really have to be achieved, will change. Diabetics who want to do well will have to change.

Medication I prescribe also helps, but a pill can't fix what you put in your mouth. A pill is the most potent example that what you put in your mouth can affect the way you feel. Eventually, you will only feel as good as you eat. My diabetic patients who do well, know this.

The rest of the book fills in the nitty-gritty but gradually, so that you can better understand and remember. I give you choices that help you individualize your own personal goals. I encourage you to spend no more than fifteen to thirty minutes a day on this diet, but to do it every day. Improve gradually. Be sure to read or reread at least 1 to 2 chapters every day. A little practice every day is more effective then one big practice per month. Repetition aids retention. Practice, one small step at a time, makes perfection.

The book also has "TEN STEPS." Completing one STEP takes usually more than 2 chapters.

I am the physician who created the "*TEN STEPS to Control Diabetes*" my patients follow. The "TEN STEPS" have been included in this book. None of these "STEPS" should be done without physician supervision and

STEP 1

advice. Some goals in STEP 1 is only for patients diagnosed by a physician as having Diabetes Mellitus Type 2 and glucotoxicity. If you are a patient (not a physician), you should not be making this diagnosis. (If you don't know what "glucotoxicity" is, that's OK, you don't need to know.)

My diabetic patients have done extremely well with this material. More than half have normal blood glucose (80-120) after more than four years. There are no results reported by doctors or researchers in the world that are better than these. I know that this material (*TEN STEPS to Control Diabetes*) helps.

It gets even better. Hypoglycemia ("low sugar") is rare in my practice. I have many patients who have maintained their weight loss and diabetes for more than eight years with this program. Few quit. All slip up at times (nobody is perfect). But many feel their best in years and that is what gets them back in step. They are just ordinary people, just like you and me. The difference for them is in this book. (Their praise and success encouraged me to write this book.)

If your doctor is unwilling to help you complete these TEN STEPS towards the control of diabetes, do not do them on your own. All the remaining chapters can still help you learn how to control your diabetes. Many patients do well without completing all the STEPS, and many complete the STEPS out of sequence. To each his own. One idea does not fit all.

Hopefully your physician will be willing to help you complete these STEPS. But if not, you can still further your cause. Eat to live, rather than live to eat. Read on, one small chapter (or two, three...) at a time.

Recommended reading for physicians:

Meijer, M. E. "An unusual approach to achieving glycemic control," *Cortlandt Forum* (September 2004): 45-48.

---

3. When You Run Out of Gas, You Run Out of Go

Trees produce the oxygen we breathe. It takes the power of the sun (light), water, and carbon dioxide for plants to grow and also produce fuel. Some of this fuel the plant uses and some of it is stored (as carbohydrates). The garden of life is powered by the sun.

When we eat plants, or animals that eat plants, we convert this food into fuel we can use. The body's fuel is glucose. The body can burn fuel (glucose) without producing flame.

However, just like a wood fire, air needs to be added to burn fuel. That's why we breathe, so we need oxygen to burn fuel (like wood). We need plants for fuel and air. When we burn glucose or wood, this fuel is converted back into carbon dioxide and water, which then can be used by plants, with the help of the sun, to make more fuel. Pretty neat!

The circle of life turns with fuel, water, and air, but is powered by the sun. All people are solar powered?

Why burn fuel? A car burns gas to work. You need energy to work. In fact, car fuel comes from the same food we use (plants). Fossil fuels are from plants and oil is used to run your car... All cars are solar powered?

People are made up of many cells. All cells are like little motors. To operate, they need energy; to get energy, they burn fuel.

Fuel, like air, is essential for life. If I choke you so that you cannot breathe, you will die from the lack of oxygen. The same result would occur if I cut off fuel instead of air. Both fuel and air keep cells in your body alive. Lacking either fuel or air, you go out like a light. Eventually, after enough of your cells stop working, you die.

A car's carburetor takes small amounts of fuel at a time and mixes it with the right amount of air. This mixture is given to the motor to burn. Burning fuel produces the energy needed to make the car go.

An old, potbellied stove has a carburetor, too. You control the amount of wood and air that goes to the fire. If all air vents are closed, there is no fire. No wood, no fire. The right mixture of both air and wood gives you the best fire.

STEP 1

The body's carburetor is the hormone insulin. Insulin is produced by cells in an organ called the pancreas (it is next to the liver). Insulin serves as a messenger, telling many other cells what to do. Insulin tells the whole body of cells how to mix fuel with air.

Like a car, we need a gas tank to store fuel. Our body stores fuel all over the place. The car has a fuel line that brings gas from the tank to the motor. Our fuel line is the circulating blood. Blood delivers fuel and oxygen to every cell in the body. Insulin in the blood controls the mixture. Too much or too little fuel makes any motor (including the body) operate poorly.

Hypoglycemia is when blood glucose (sugar) is too low. Low gas, slow go. Mild hypoglycemia causes weakness. Severe hypoglycemia can result in coma. No go for good means you're dead.

Hypoglycemia is caused by too much insulin or not enough fuel. Blood glucose is the fuel that makes you go. If you want to keep going, don't run out of gas. Hyperglycemia (high blood glucose levels) defines diabetes. But diabetics can also get hypoglycemia (low blood glucose levels). A better definition of diabetes is bad blood glucose control. Diabetes is like having a motor without a carburetor (or one that is broken).

A motor with a flooded carburetor runs very poorly or not at all. A wood stove with too much wood and not enough air also burns poorly or not at all. A correct mixture of fuel and air is very important.

Hyperglycemia (high sugar) is caused by too much food, not enough insulin, or by cells in the body that do not respond to insulin as they should. Imagine if you had a car with an engine that did not have a carburetor. To make the motor run, you would have to spoon-feed the right amount of fuel into the engine continuously. If you dumped a whole bunch of fuel at once, you would flood the engine and then later (down the road), you would run out of gas. If you got lazy and just stopped feeding the motor, it would stop running.

When food is eaten, blood glucose (sugar) rises. Eating infrequently with large meals will "flood" the blood stream with glucose (fuel). In between big meals, running out of gas could be a problem. If you skip too many meals, you run out of gas. If you eat too much fuel (food) all day, your "engine" that makes you go stays flooded all day.

Some people without known diabetes can also develop hypoglycemia. The more food one eats, the more insulin one needs to control blood glucose. Extra insulin is normally produced to make blood glucose levels fall. But too much insulin can then cause hypoglycemia.

People who have trouble with hypoglycemia can also run out of gas if they don't fill the tank (skip too many meals).

The best way to prevent hypoglycemia is to eat frequently in small amounts. "A little of a lot rather than a lot of a little." This is also the best way to treat or prevent hyperglycemia (which is diabetes).

The symptoms of hypoglycemia include weakness, severe hunger, light-headedness, excess sweating, nervousness, confusion, irritability, and passing out. The motor either stops or sputters. No go for good means you are dead. Hypoglycemia is very dangerous.

The easiest way to turn off a motor is to turn off the fuel. It's harder to turn off the motor by giving it too much gas.

It takes severe hyperglycemia to put a diabetic into a coma. Normally all hyperglycemia does is make diabetics feel bad (your flooded motor runs like crap). Diabetics with frequent high blood glucose levels feel like crap. You can only feel as good as you eat.

In other words, it's easier to starve to death than it is to eat to death...*but both can be done.* Don't skip needed meals. Don't overeat.

It also should be easy to understand that a motor needs the right kind of fuel (quality). A gasoline motor cannot run on diesel fuel.

Another dietary aid to prevent both hypo- and hyperglycemia is to eat high-fiber, quality foods. It's believed that fiber slows the absorption of fuel from food, but this has never been well-proven. Regardless of how fiber works, it has been proven that a high-fiber diet prevents both hypoglycemia and hyperglycemia.

Patients who suffer from hypoglycemia or from diabetes can easily appreciate the importance of a good diet. A diet is everything you put into

Step 1

your mouth. There is no insulin shot or pill that can overcome too many or too few calories. A pill can't make chicken salad out of chicken crap. You can only feel as good as you eat.

In order for a motor to run well, it needs the correct amount (quantity) of high-fiber food (quality) delivered continuously. Quantity of fuel in food is measured in calories. Most junk food ("crap") is low in fiber and high in calories. A high fiber, low calorie diet tends to improve the kinds of food most Americans would eat, not just how much. A high fiber diet is a quality diet. Both quantity and quality are important. One can neither fast nor feast, but what you eat matters too.

It is carefully measured caloric intake and six small meals a day that keep a body without a carburetor "running" properly. Patients, especially diabetics, feel and live as good as they eat. Proper fuel (quantity & quality) intake (diet) becomes a matter of life and death. You either grow old or die young, those are your choices.

But when you run out of gas, you run out of go.

4. Update on Diabetes Mellitus

The ancient Greeks observed that some patients began to urinate excessively. They also noticed that a large number of flies were attracted to the urine. Tasting the urine, it was found to be sweeter than normal. It was concluded that the loss of this sweet substance was the underlying cause of this disease. Once this sweet substance was detected in the urine, the patients then wasted away and died, some much more rapidly than others. The Greek word *diabetes* means "a siphon." The Greek word *melitos* means "honey." We now know this "honey" is glucose. The "newer" Latin word currently used is Diabetes Mellitus.

Diabetes itself has not changed; only our knowledge has. The words we use, including definitions, have also changed (as recommended by the American Diabetic Association, i.e. ADA). The ways we diagnose diabetes have changed too. Fortunately for doctors, we don't have to taste the urine anymore.

Not all patients have the same diabetes. We know about two "flavors" of diabetes. They are now cleverly named, using the new terminology of the ADA, Diabetes Mellitus Type 1 (DM Type 1) and Diabetes Mellitus Type 2 (DM Type 2). In the recent past, the Roman numerals I & II were used, but this has been updated. DM Type 1 and DM Type 2 are actually two different diseases. Most diabetics are Type 2. It is a modern medical triumph, made possible by the discovery of insulin, that so many diabetics are still alive. Since patients now survive with this disorder, diabetes has become more common. Patients might not feel blessed by being diagnosed with diabetes. Agreed, but it is a blessing that patients can now control their disease *if they so choose.*

DM Type 1 patients have a rapid rise in blood glucose level (sugar) with the onset of this disease. They usually get sick very fast. Unlike DM Type 2, there is very little delay in diagnosing DM Type 1. There is little delay in beginning insulin treatment. DM Type 1 diabetics stop producing needed insulin. Insulin is a hormone. Hormones are produced by one type of cells to

Step 1

tell other cells in our bodies what to do.

When compared to DM Type 2, controlling blood glucose is more difficult in DM Type 1. In the past, DM Type 1 was called "Brittle" Diabetes, or more commonly, Insulin Dependent Diabetes Mellitus (IDDM). The ADA no longer recommends using these words. This is because eventually all diabetics need insulin (including Type 2).

Remember DM Type 1 and DM Type 2 are two different diseases. In DM Type 1, insulin is no longer produced. In DM Type 2, cells of the body that are supposed to listen to insulin, **don't**. This problem is called Insulin Resistance.

Initially, when cells don't listen well, the pancreas (the organ that makes insulin) starts yelling (i.e. makes more insulin). This stage of DM Type 2 begins 10-15 years before blood glucose ("sugar") rises. The increased production of insulin can overcome and maintain normal or almost-normal blood glucose levels for those many years. The ten to fifteen years of excessive yelling (i.e. high levels of insulin) damage many parts of the body. The harm caused by DM Type 2 begins when insulin resistance develops (i.e. excessive production of insulin starts), not when elevated blood glucose finally begins to rise. We can treat insulin resistance. Therefore, any delay in diagnosis of DM Type 2 causes preventable harm from high insulin levels. Eventually, the pancreas in Type 2 diabetics becomes "hoarse." Extra insulin production can no longer keep up with the body's added demand for insulin. Then diabetes overtly develops, relatively speaking, by a shortage of insulin. Only then does blood glucose rise. Eventually, insulin production completely fails (ends) and the Type 2 diabetic finally needs insulin.

Diabetes Type 1 begins as a totally different problem. This diabetes is caused by the lack of insulin. This is because the cells in the pancreas that make insulin are mistakenly destroyed by the immune system. Why this happens, we do not know.

Prevention or earlier treatment for DM Type 1 will depend on genetic research. Our genes control our immune system. It is speculated that environmental events (such as a cold virus) can cause our genes to react in a

Step 1

way that causes DM Type 1. It is hoped that genetic research can find a way to stop the immune system from destroying the pancreas. Another option for cure is to replace the lost insulin-producing cells with genetic engineering. This, too, is being looked into.

A significant advance in the treatment of DM Type 1 is the very expensive insulin pump. This is not for everyone. Insulin pumps provide a variable but continuous infusion of insulin to control blood sugar. Small malfunctions can be very dangerous. Pumps are rarely used for Type 2 DM.

Usually the beginning treatment for DM Type 2 is **not** insulin. Most people are familiar with the fact that there are "pills" that treat diabetes. These old pills worked by helping the pancreas produce more insulin (i.e. even more "yelling"). Eventually, this strategy always failed. The pancreas would again lose its voice. Insulin production would not be adequate.

Research has produced new drugs that make cells listen better to insulin. This is an obvious improvement over older pills available for DM Type 2 patients. Even when insulin shots are needed, less insulin is required. The only problem with the new medication is cost. These drugs are expensive.

The wonderful ability to treat what was normally a fatal disease with pills and insulin has led the general public to believe that this is the only treatment needed for diabetes. This is not true. Just as important is dietary therapy. **Failure to improve diet undermines all other treatments for diabetes.** In fact, a bad diet and obesity can dramatically increase (60 fold or more) your chances to develop DM Type 2. Currently, one in five Americans can expect to develop diabetes. As obesity rises, this number will increase, too.

Abnormal blood glucose levels needed to diagnose DM Type 2 have been lowered by the new ADA guidelines for diabetes. A normal fasting (nothing to eat or drink overnight) blood level is from 80-120. The new fasting blood glucose level recommended to diagnose diabetes is one greater than 126. Some patients in the past have been told they had "borderline diabetes". These patients are no longer considered borderline. You either have diabetes or you don't. You just might not know it.

The ADA now recommends that physicians screen and counsel patients who are at high risk to develop DM Type 2 (not Type 1). These risk factors include a family history of DM Type 2, obesity, evidence of early hypertension (high blood pressure), history of gestational diabetes (abnormal blood glucose levels during pregnancy), polycystic ovary syndrome, some lipid/cholesterol abnormalities, etc...(see your doctor). It has been proven that early dietary changes with or without medication can prevent blood glucose from ever rising to levels diagnostic for DM type 2. By starting treatment in these patients much sooner than before, problems normally caused by DM Type 2 might even be prevented.

The fatal outcome of untreated Diabetes Mellitus is adequately described by the ancient Greeks. Both types of diabetes are bad. All diabetic patients are at risk for kidney failure (dialysis), amputation, blindness, strokes, heart attacks, sudden death, congestive heart failure, impotence, infertility, pulmonary embolus (blood clots in the lung), polyneuropathy (diffuse burning, pain, and/or numbness of extremities), senile dementia, and susceptibility to all kinds of dangerous infections (ask your doctor). These problems can be slowed or prevented with early and aggressive treatment for diabetes. Paramount to this is improved diet. For many DM Type 2 patients, this means losing weight as well.

Our knowledge and advice changes, Diabetes does not. We know you can live well if you want to. Neglect Diabetes, history will always repeat itself.

5. Progressive Disease, Sudden Problems

Many diseases are not discovered at their onset. Rather, illness becomes apparent after many years of disease. Knowing you have a disease and having a disease are two different things.

Arthritis is a classic example. The gradual wear and tear of joints goes unnoticed. One day, a joint suddenly hurts and swells. Arthritis is "discovered." Once arthritis has progressed enough that symptoms have developed, symptoms can persist (wax and wane). It's the "straw that broke the camel's back" that made arthritis noticeable.

Many diseases can be detected before symptoms develop if deliberately looked for. Not all of these diseases are treatable. It makes no sense to detect a disease early that you cannot treat. Screening for early problems only makes sense if early intervention can make a difference down the road. Recommendations for screening tests are made with this in mind. However, most patients don't want to be bothered looking for unnoticed diseases.

Out of sight, out of mind. It's human nature to ignore information; we do this every day. When listening to someone talk, our brain automatically filters out any background noise. When looking at a small object, the eyeball sees much more than the brain sees. Our thoughts only "see" the object of interest. You can try this yourself. If you deliberately listen for background noise, you will notice more sounds than originally heard. While looking at an object, deliberately pay attention to the edge of your vision. You will see much more than you did before.

The body's capacity to see and hear is more than what we usually need. We ignore what we don't use. Loss of hearing is noticed when it interferes with understanding speech. The prior loss of background noise goes undetected.

The lung's ability to deliver oxygen exceeds normal demands. Disease can destroy this reserve lung capacity. Lung disease is only noticed when oxygen demands are not met and you become unusually short of breath. But while there is loss of unused lung, no shortness of breath will develop, and this loss goes undetected. People with noticeable shortness of breath from lung disease have already had more than half of their lungs completely destroyed. Once lung reserves are marginal, any slight further loss of lung function or increased demand for air becomes extremely noticeable. You are either short of breath or you are not. Most lung diseases have developed slowly and unnoticed. (Of course, there are some lung diseases that can develop quickly.) This occurs because it is the large and unused lung reserve capacity that has been gradually destroyed. In sharp contrast, the onset of shortness of breath is usually very sudden.

Walking on a frozen pond is no problem until the ice breaks. When a frozen pond thaws, thick ice doesn't suddenly become thin. Ice melts gradually. No matter how dangerously thin the ice is, it's not a problem as long as it doesn't break and you're still walking. Falling through ice into a frozen pond is dangerous (life threatening). There is no in-between. You are either in the water or out. The process (thinning ice) is gradual. The problem is sudden (drowning).

Many medical problems take years to develop. A person can be totally unaware how thin the ice is that they are standing on. Worse yet, the time between cracks developing and the ice breaking can be very short. You can suddenly become very ill.

Most lung diseases occur in smokers. The disease can be anticipated. Pulmonary function tests (breathing tests) crudely measure lung capacity and function. Early disease can still be missed, but lung disease can be detected using breathing tests long before shortness of breath develops. Ample warning can usually be given to those who choose to look and/or listen.

Heart disease can easily be missed with many heart tests. However, risk factors, such as high blood pressure, can make heart disease likely. Therefore, preventive treatment can be started without evidence of actual heart disease. The likelihood of high blood pressure causing heart disease may be reason enough to take an aspirin-a-day, etc.

Unfortunately many diseases detected early are ignored, as long as no symptoms have developed, by patients. High blood pressure has no symptoms. When early disease has no ill consequences (i.e. no headache), it can be neglected without obvious problems. A patient cannot compare the current inconvenience of treatment (e.g., cost, changes in diet, etc...) with the future inconvenience of disease (a stroke or heart attack that has not yet occurred). Human nature finds it easy to look only at what can be obviously seen or heard — the current inconvenience of treatment or preventive care.

Imagine how hard it would be to convince people who have stood on ice their entire life how dangerous thin ice can be. Remember, for many people, the ice has never been thin enough to fall through (i.e. they have never really been sick). While standing on the thin ice — there is absolutely no difference between thick ice and thin ice. You're still well and dry. There is also no guarantee that the thinner ice will actually break.

Doctors face this every day. It is very difficult to convince people that the ice can break before it does break.

Also remember, some people drown when the ice breaks. Not everyone gets a second chance (to be well and dry). Even though there are circumstances where ice breaks for no apparent reason, many drownings are predictable.

Common diseases occur commonly (that's common sense).

Uncontrolled and/or untreated high blood glucose will predictably and gradually kill cells in your body. These losses go unnoticed until enough cells are killed that make you suddenly face serious problems.

Problems caused by high blood glucose include blindness, dialysis, and amputations. Maintaining normal sugar control (even if you have diabetes) will stop these losses of cells. But remember, it can be too late once the ice breaks.

Screening tests for diseases can be tried on people who have a good chance of having any disease. Screening tests are usually more helpful if done before disease becomes evident (you still feel well)). Tests are selected based on age, sex, family history of disease, personal living habits, and costs. Obviously, screening to prevent disease or to detect disease early should be highly individualized.

When's the last time you had a complete physical?

Most Americans take better care of their car.

STEP 1

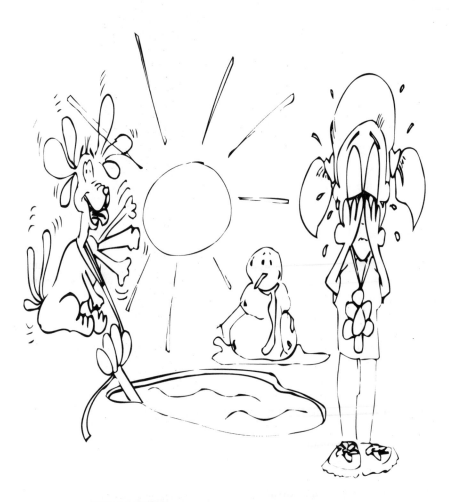

WARM ENOUGH?

Step 1

6. Understanding Diet for Control of Diabetes

Diabetes Mellitus (DM) is more often called "high sugar." It is a disease where the body no longer controls sugar (glucose) in the blood properly.

Glucose is the body's fuel. Every cell in the body is like a little engine. In order for the engine to run correctly, it needs fuel and air. In the body, blood brings glucose and oxygen to every cell. The blood picks up the oxygen from the lungs and it gets the glucose (fuel) from cells that store glucose and from the stomach (when we are eating).

Everyone understands that they will die if their heart stops beating. This is because the blood stops circulating to all the cells. All living cells stop working and die when they are no longer supplied with air and fuel (oxygen and glucose).

By far the most important "engine" in the body is the brain. If brain cells do not receive either oxygen or glucose, they stop working and die. Irreversible brain death occurs in about ten to fifteen minutes. Therefore, it is a matter of life and death that all cells receive both oxygen and a good supply of glucose.

The body has many systems designed to try to prevent death. If you are knocked unconscious, you will continue to breathe by an automatic system despite the fact you are "out cold."

Since glucose is so important, the body has many ways to prevent sugar from becoming too low. However, there are fewer systems built into the body to prevent sugar from becoming too high. When the body's system that controls the blood sugar is broken (which is diabetes), it is much more likely that the sugar is too high rather than too low. But while a diabetic's primary problem is that his sugar is too high, low sugar can also be a problem. So really Diabetes Mellitus is a disease where the blood sugar is out of control, not just "high sugar."

Insulin is a hormone produced by an organ called the pancreas. Digested food is converted into glucose (fuel). Insulin tells cells what to do with

Step 1

glucose. It's not practical for a person to eat food constantly. It makes sense that the body has a system for energy storage (gas tank).

Some glucose is transported and "put in storage" (fat and muscle). Some is used immediately. Stored glucose can later be released and transported for use. The transportation and use of glucose is controlled and coordinated by insulin. Insulin provides the communication needed between cells throughout the body to ensure a good fuel supply in the blood stream. When cells no longer respond to insulin or when there is no insulin to respond to, communication between cells breaks down. If cells do not "hear" insulin, blood glucose levels will be "out of control." This is diabetes.

Type 1 diabetics do not make insulin at all. Without any insulin, blood glucose has to quickly rise. However, most diabetics suffer from "insulin resistance." This is called Diabetes Type 2.

The cells of Type 2 diabetics no longer respond properly to insulin (no longer "listen"). Initially, the pancreas compensates for this by making more and more insulin (e.g., yelling). Eventually, not enough insulin can be produced to overcome "insulin resistance." Then blood glucose rises.

It's the job of the kidneys to remove undesired substances from the bloodstream so that it can be eliminated. The kidneys also have to keep in what we need. It makes sense that the kidneys would try to keep glucose from being eliminated. However, the kidneys' capacity to do their job can be exceeded. Excessively high blood glucose levels exceed the capacity of the kidneys to keep the glucose in the blood. When this happens, sugar spills out into the urine. Diabetics with uncontrolled sugar urinate their fuel away. This wasted fuel (glucose) can exceed our ability to eat and drink. It also exceeds our bodies' ability to use stored glucose from fat. Fuel (glucose) for high energy demands is provided by breaking down muscle, rather than fat. Therefore, uncontrolled diabetics lose their muscle mass, not fat, when blood glucose is too high. Uncontrolled diabetics run out of gas. (It is flushed down the toilet.) Eventually, dehydrated and comatose, the uncontrolled diabetic will waste away and die.

Imagine if you had a car with an engine that did not have a carbure-

STEP 1

tor. Remember, a motor works by burning fuel mixed with air. Fuel needs oxygen to burn just like a wood fire. The carburetor, for those who don't know, mixes the right amount of fuel and air. It then feeds this mixture slowly to the engine. Too much fuel in the mixture and the engine "floods" (it may clog up and not start, or it simply doesn't run well). With too little fuel, the motor will run out of gas and stop. If you were given a car with no carburetor, to make it run you would have to spoon feed the right amount of fuel into the engine continuously. If you dumped a whole bunch of fuel in at once, you would flood the engine and then later (down the road) you would run out of gas.

A diabetic has a similar problem. Their "carburetors" don't work well. Insulin is the carburetor for the body. It controls how fuel mixes in the body. Eating infrequently with large meals (like our traditional three meals a day) will "flood" the bloodstream with glucose (fuel). In between big meals, running out of gas could be a problem. If you eat too much fuel (food) all day, the engine stays flooded all day. If you skip too many meals, you run out of gas.

A continuous level of properly measured glucose with oxygen must be maintained in the blood. If this is to be maintained when the "carburetor" is broken, food (fuel) needs to be "spoon fed" throughout the day. Diabetics need to "spoon feed" themselves with frequent, small meals. How much fuel there is in food is measured in calories. The correct amount of food (measured in calories) needs to be eaten at each small meal. Both when and how many calories is important. Activity levels will also determine how much food (fuel) is needed (a motor wide open takes more fuel than one that is just idling). No diabetic can do well without a proper diet. There is no insulin shot or any other medication that can overcome too many or too few calories. Your "diet" is everything **you** put in your mouth.

I hope you begin to realize how important a diabetic's diet is to help control blood glucose. It not only needs to be nutritionally balanced, it needs to be the right amount of "gas" (calories) at the right times.

One can neither fast nor feast.

Step 1

Rather, it is a carefully measured caloric intake and six small meals a day that help keep the diabetic's body "running" properly. Every cell (motor) in the body is affected by glucose control. Diabetics feel and live as well as they eat. Proper fuel intake (**diet!**) for a diabetic is a matter of life and death.

You run out of gas, you run out of go.

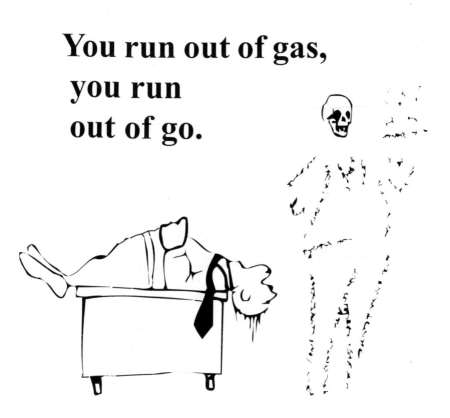

7. Lowering Resistance to Diabetes (Type 2)

We have talked about the importance of the diabetic diet (i.e. calories) for the treatment of Diabetes Mellitus. Without proper diet, you eventually cannot control diabetes. It is a matter of life and death for a diabetic to maintain glucose control.

Digested food is changed into glucose. This "fuel" is measured in calories. Excessive energy (calories) has to be stored. Insulin tells fat cells to take glucose from the blood stream and convert it into fat (fat cells get bigger). Excessive calories combined with excessive insulin (e.g., DM Type 2) result in more body fat (obesity). The liver converts food into the smallest, most elementary, energy-carrying compound found in the body (glucose). Insulin tells liver cells to stop putting glucose into the blood. Insulin also tells muscle cells to absorb the glucose needed to contract the muscles that make you go. Insulin lowers blood glucose levels.

If insulin is absent *or* when cells don't "listen" to insulin (i.e. insulin resistance), the liver puts out too much glucose. Fat and muscle cells can't use the excess glucose. Blood glucose levels can only go up. The great irony here is that, despite high levels of fuel in the blood supply, all cells are limited in their ability to use glucose as needed (due to insulin resistance). No wonder uncontrolled diabetes makes people feel sick and tired. Excessive insulin in Diabetes Type 2, not just glucose, causes damage. The ideal way to treat diabetes is to also lower the amount of insulin needed to control glucose.

One way to lower the amounts of insulin needed per day is to just not overeat. Simple, isn't it? In addition, the more you eat (calories) at one time, the more your sugar level can also rise. The higher the glucose blood level, the more insulin you will need to lower those sugar levels. Frequent small meals solve this problem.

High fiber foods and complex carbohydrates (e.g., fruit, etc.) take longer for the body to dissolve and digest (i.e. convert these foods into blood glucose). Sugar (e.g., sodas) is the exact opposite. It is a small molecule that is broken down quickly into glucose. It is absorbed immediately by the body.

Step 1

Glucose from sugar then rushes into the blood stream, resulting in a sudden high level of glucose. With sodas, you get a "sugar high" in the blood stream requiring a sudden increase in circulating insulin to bring it down.

In DM Type 2 with "insulin resistance," the cells of the body do not listen well to insulin. Sudden demands for changes by insulin are responded to very slowly. This again results in high glucose levels. The consequences of this is that the body needs more insulin to deal with the "sugar high." More insulin and more high blood glucose means more cell damage (such as kidney cells, nerve cells, etc.). It's a vicious cycle.

Many people are now aware of fat grams. The problem with food that has a high fat content is that it also has a high calorie content. In order to digest food, the body converts fat to glucose. One cup of lard equals four cups of sugar. So the diabetic who eats fatty foods easily eats too many calories. A fatty meal also results in a high spike of sugar since a small amount of fat holds four times more sugar (glucose) than ordinary foods (such as bread and other carbohydrates).

Well-controlled sugar—that is, well-maintained, normal blood glucose—will lower insulin resistance. The more poorly-controlled sugar—that is, "high sugar"—the higher your insulin resistance will be. Higher insulin resistance causes even higher blood glucose levels (which in turn, increases insulin resistance). We know this to be true. This is a vicious cycle in terms of trying to control diabetes.

So the higher your blood glucose levels are every day, the more you need insulin. As people who take insulin shots will tell you, the higher the sugar levels are, the more insulin the doctor must add to the shots. Again, it's a vicious cycle.

Obesity—a high number of fat cells in your body—increases insulin resistance. Simply put, the fatter you are, the harder it is to control your blood glucose (e.g., diabetes). The only solution is **DIET**. If you are overweight (five or more pounds) and a diabetic, you need to lose weight. Losing five pounds can cut insulin resistance in half for DM Type 2 (*WOW!*).

In contrast, lean body mass requires less insulin, and therefore glucose in the blood is easier to control. Exercise is extremely helpful in lowering weight. In addition, exercised and well-conditioned muscles need less insulin, which again lowers insulin resistance.

There are many medicines, which folks call "sugar pills," to control diabetes. Some of these medications lower insulin resistance (they are not all the same). These newer drugs make the cells of the body more responsive to insulin. This in turn lowers glucose levels.

Diabetes will get worse over time (you get older). Unfortunately, for DM Type 2, the pancreas eventually burns itself out when making excessive insulin. Sooner or later, if a diabetic lives long enough, he or she will need insulin.

Adding insulin to the patient's medicine increases the amount of circulating insulin, which in turn, damages cells in the body. However, failure to control sugar can kill you as well. Very high blood glucose will put you in a coma and can cause death in hours. The lesser of two evils is to add insulin therapy.

Bottom line: when you need to start insulin, you *NEED* to start insulin. There is no way around it. But you still want to do everything you can to lower your insulin resistance and use as little insulin as possible. And that brings us right back to diet and weight control, diet and exercise, and diet and diet.

The evidence is overwhelming that most diabetics can learn to control blood glucose levels to such a degree that normal blood sugar levels can be maintained. Those diabetics watch their diets continuously—**no** ifs, ands, or buts. Insulin resistance can also be lowered. These diabetics greatly reduce harm to their bodies caused by these two problems. A diabetic with normal (that is, very good) sugar control can have a nearly-normal life expectancy.

Either the diabetic controls his/her glucose or glucose controls the diabetic. Eventually high blood glucose forces the diabetic into either the hospital very sick or into the funeral home. So, if you are a diabetic, you have to decide which kind you want to be:

(a) the kind who controls blood sugar, feels good, and can expect to

STEP 1

enjoy a good life by following the needed diet
OR
(b) the kind who lives only to eat, lets blood sugar get out of control, feels badly all the time, and shortens his/her life.
You'll feel as good as you eat.

WHICH **BOAT** WOULD YOU RATHER **BE ON?**

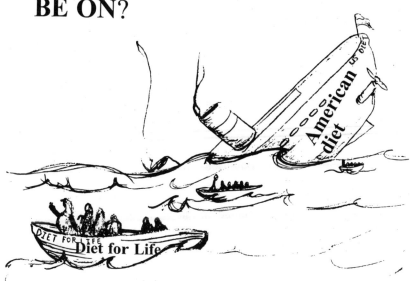

8. How to Use TEN STEPS to Control Diabetes

Some of our diabetic patients do so well that after a while, they forget they are diabetic! Some simply want to forget. Since most diabetics have to make and maintain difficult dietary changes, I find it wise to leave no doubt about the diagnosis of diabetes. At the first office visit, I always made sure diabetic patients are convinced that their diagnosis was diabetes.

The first STEP is designed for newly diagnosed glucotoxic Type 2 diabetics. The 1st STEP involves a three-day fast which ends in three days or when blood glucose falls below 130mg/dl (whichever comes first). Fasting can also be used on Type 2 diabetics who are on medications but have become glucotoxic. I generally maintain those medications during the fast but blood glucose has to be more carefully monitored.

The science of fasting is old. Before the discovery of insulin, it was the only treatment available. No one starves to death in three days.

In the 1970s, fasting was researched and used extensively. If you want a comprehensive, modern, college-level, medical textbook on Diabetes, that discusses fasting, I recommend *Clinical Diabetes Mellitus, a Problem Approach*. Medical literature references are included. The 3rd edition was copyrighted in 2000. It is published by THIEME. You can order this book from their web site.

Of course, if you can understand a "comprehensive, modern, college-level, medical textbook," you probably wouldn't be reading this book. I provide this reference so that you can tell your health care provider(s) what to read if they have questions about fasting diabetics.

The author, John K. Davidson, MD, was himself a diabetic. He was also a Boarded Endocrinologist, Professor of Medicine, and an accomplished researcher. Now retired, his successful treatment protocols have been ignored or forgotten by most younger physicians. I use a modified approach. Dr. Davidson used a seven day fast, I use three days or less. He stopped using all oral medications, I do not. He hospitalized patients for the duration of the fast, I do not. Type 1 diabetics were also made to fast, I do not recom-

Step 1

mend Type 1 diabetics fast.

A three-day fast, properly supervised, is extremely safe. I am unaware of any reported deaths for a three-day fast. Deaths due to starvation have been reported in very sick patients who have fasted for seven days or more. The safety of a three-day fast was one reason I chose a three-day fast over a seven-day one. But even a seven-day fast, properly supervised, is very safe and medically sound for properly selected diabetic patients.

The next chapter is the first "STEP" (STEP 1) of ten steps I use with many of my patients. It is a close reproduction of the patient education handout I give my patients at the end of their first office visit. Obviously, my handouts correspond with what I do and say during the visit. There is no right or wrong way to precisely do these steps, this is just an example of my way.

I write and give my own patient education handouts so my patients can avoid complex advice from the American Diabetic Association (ADA). Important differences exist between my material and that provided by the ADA. The most obvious is STEP 1, which includes my use of a three-day fast.

Previous National Institute of Health (NIH) consensus panels acknowledged the effective use of fasting for the treatment of diabetes, but current ones do not. The reason for this is unknown. ADA politics, I'm sure, played an important role.

The other obvious difference I have with the ADA is that I do not like most of their patient education material. Their current scientific babble (which they always refer to as "patient education") has confused more patients than ever before. Some "patient education" seems very self-serving. I am concerned the ADA may be more interested in getting my patients to help them (by sending them money) than helping my diabetics treat their disease.

While under the "leadership" of the ADA, the epidemic of diabetes Type 2 in America has become much larger. Every scientist in the world would agree that diet plays a major role in this epidemic. There is no proof that what the ADA has told the public, Congress, physicians, or patients to

Step 1

do is helping to stop this growing epidemic..

The ADA's position is that their methods/advice would work if everyone would do exactly what they are being told to do. Maybe some could if the ADA's expert advice wasn't such a large amount of mangled scientific babble and complicated "crap." It's mangled because committees produce this stuff.

Americans can't make chicken salad out of chicken crap.

My diet program doesn't do anything weird. In fact, most of the science is from the most recent one hundred years. The real difference between this program and other scientific programs is the language. I speak plain English that ordinary people can understand. Furthermore, whether you are highly educated or not, your motivation to improve your diet gets better with this program.

It's not what we say, it's how we say it.

My patients and I are not perfect, so we do the best we can do. Despite our flaws, we achieve much better results than those being reported by the followers of the ADA. My patients and I believe the Ten Steps I use are a lot clearer then the endless, expertly managed, programs associated with the ADA. This clarity of goals set by *Ten Steps to Control Diabetes* is the reason for our success. Remember, some of those "experts" went to the same medical school I went to. So who has determined that they are better than any other doctor? They did! I encourage you to simply read on, one clear step at a time, and judge for yourself.

9. *STEP 1* for Control of Diabetes

The FIRST STEP to staying alive is to stop killing yourself with bad food. A bad diet is not worth dying for. Changing the way you eat is "life and death." A new diet for a new life. Today is the first day for the rest of your life. If you so choose, today is the first step toward *your control* over diabetes.

Goals for STEP 1:
Be sure you understand the 4 chapters about diabetes:

    4. Update on Diabetes Mellitus
    6. Understanding Diet for Control of Diabetes
    7. Lowering Resistance to Diabetes
    5. Progressive Disease, Sudden Problems

Everything you need to know, for now, about diabetes is in these four chapters (this is just the first step). *6. Understanding Diet for Control of Diabetes* is the most important chapter to understand (learn it!).

You probably have heard that diet is important for treating diabetes. The first step for **glucotoxicity (diagnosed by a physician)** is a diet that is very simple and easy to understand — **Don't eat anything** (you will not starve to death in 3 days).

Do not eat until one of these two things happen:

    1) *three (3) days have passed (72 hours);* **OR**
    2) your blood glucose (sugar) has fallen to 130 or less.

You can check your sugar in three different ways. You can ask your doctor to prescribe a glucometer so you can check your "sugars" (blood glucose levels) on your own. You can ask a friend or family member (who is a diabetic or nurse) to check it for you with their machine. You can see a doctor or nurse daily and let them check it.

When you resume eating, eat sensibly and less.

If fasting, drink water and diet sodas, no juices. In the next step you will need to stop drinking diet sodas (i.e. ALL sodas). If you are not already drinking diet sodas, don't start. Take a once-a-day multivitamin (the cheapest one you find is okay).

STEP 1

Questions commonly asked by patients:

Are you sure I have diabetes? Our office repeats at least two (2) tests on two separate blood samples (checked four times). We diagnose diabetes in three different ways. If you have any doubts that you have diabetes, let your doctor know on your next visit.

What is a normal (fasting) blood glucose level? It is 100+ 20 (80-120).

Will I be prescribed medicine for diabetes? Yes. Even with normal sugars, we no longer treat diabetes by diet alone. But diet is still the most important treatment for diabetes. Diet is your first prescribed treatment for diabetes.

Why do I have to read all this paperwork given to me? What you don't know can still hurt you. You can't do well ignoring your diabetes. Untreated and ignored, diabetes is fatal. No one can do for you what you must do for yourself. No one can breathe for you, no one can eat for you, no one can learn for you. You must know what you have. You need to learn how to take care of diabetes.

Do I really have to change the way I eat? Only if you want to live.

How can I learn all this stuff at one time? You can't. You will learn "all this stuff" one step at a time. Some of this "stuff" is really boring. Read a few chapters every day, but do it EVERYDAY. It took years for your doctor to learn all this. He didn't learn it all at once either. You will go to the next step when you have completed (and learned) this step. Don't get ahead of us or yourself. Learn this step well, then we will move on to the next step.

I have heard (or seen) that diabetes can cause bad things — will this happen to me? It doesn't have to. If you work really hard (are you a hard worker?), you can achieve normal sugars and eliminate the harm high sugars can cause. Go read the chapters over and over again until you know them well. If you are ready by the next office visit, you can proceed to the next step.

STEP 1

What bad things can happen to me now that I have diabetes? Ask your doctor about any particular thing that might worry you. Do you know someone who has diabetes who is having problems? Write it down so you won't forget to ask about any special worries.

Questions your doctor might ask you:
> *Do you want to live?*
> *Will you learn the diet?*
> *Did you complete Step One?*
> *Do you know all your medication bottles?*
> *Do you have any questions, concerns, or problems?*

Modern medicine's ability to treat diabetes with pills and insulin has led some people to believe that this is the **only** treatment needed for diabetes. It's **not.** Failure to improve diet undermines **all** other treatments for diabetes. The **first** treatment for diabetes must be **diet.**

Step 2

10. Why the Big Fuss?

One physician said, *"Obesity and inactivity are an epidemic in the U.S. of such disastrous proportion that it makes HIV disease look like a minor viral illness."*

Why so much fuss about losing weight? It's because obesity, lack of exercise and poor diet are connected to many diseases. It's irrelevant how much each of these factors actually contributes to disease since all three are so intertwined. It's very appropriate to say that an ounce of prevention is worth a pound of cure.

In my practice, obesity could no longer be ignored. More and more patients could no longer be weighed by my old scales. These patients exceeded the maximum measurable weight for the scales (350 pounds). In addition, an overwhelming number of my patients that could be weighed were gaining weight. It's also very worrisome to see how many children are obese.

I practiced in Aynor, SC. Most recent South Carolina statistics agree with my observations. South Carolina is ranked tenth highest in obesity in the United States. More than half of all South Carolina residents are overweight. The number of obese children has doubled in the last twenty years. Fat kids are likely to be fat adults. This has resulted in a 400% increase of Diabetes Type 2 in children. South Carolina is in fifteenth place in diabetic deaths in America. Fully 90% of diabetics are overweight.

Is diabetes common in South Carolina? You bet your belly it is!

Late intervention is never as good as early preventive care. Initially, obesity can be ignored. Eventually, obesity takes its toll. The earlier weight control begins, the earlier obesity can be avoided.

Not all preventive care has proven worthwhile. The publicity suggesting that salt reduction would reduce hypertension was greatly exaggerated. The long-term effect of excessive salt on hypertension in most patients is small.

In contrast, obesity has an enormous long-term effect on hypertension. Losing weight can cause a dramatic improvement in blood pressure

Step 2

control. But the success of medication, technology, and surgery has over-shadowed the importance of diet, exercise and weight control. (Inaccurate or misleading dietary advice has not helped, either.).

The American Cancer Society is becoming increasingly more interested in emphasizing the importance of diet. Improved diet and the reduction of obesity may reduce cancer related deaths by as much as 50%. These kinds of results are hard to ignore.

Very expensive diseases, such as diabetes, are greatly influenced by diet, exercise, and obesity. The most common diabetes is Type 2. Type 2 Diabetes runs strongly in families. But the most important reason as to whether an individual develops or does not develop diabetes is obesity and diet. The onset of damage from diabetes is estimated to be 10 years before blood sugars are elevated and the diagnosis can be made. Diabetes can be a well-kept secret. Obesity, diet, and family history are not.

Many people are amazed at the variety of complications obesity can cause. Obesity is an important cause of sleep apnea. These patients stop breathing while sleeping which, in turn, disrupts sleep with awakening. Their eyes are still closed but they are not getting restful sleep. Without restful sleep, these patients suffer from excessive sleepiness during the day. The number of people who fall asleep behind the wheel while driving is difficult to calculate but many believe this problem exceeds drunk driving as a cause of accidents. In any event, chronic fatigue destroys the quality of life and sleep apnea can cause other symptoms — such as severe headaches.

Gall bladder disease has reached record numbers in the United States. Obesity is the greatest identifiable, preventable risk factor for this problem.

A lot of heart failure can trace its origins to obesity.

Not all illnesses attributable to obesity are life-threatening. Very common problems, such as lower back pain and arthritis in the legs, are clearly made worse by obesity. Once morbid obesity develops, the ability to exercise falls. The lack of exercise makes further weight gain even more likely. These kinds of problems create vicious cycles that increase the rate of weight gain. You become fatter faster.

STEP 2

How a person looks should not matter as much as it does. The psychological toll, especially for women, on being perceived as obese and unattractive is very high. This is especially true for teenagers.

The perception that obesity is viewed as unattractive is very real. While some people find obesity attractive, the majority does not. This is reflected by lower salaries, higher unemployment and fewer promotions. The amount of suffering cannot be easily measured.

Many patients are irritated or offended by advice to lose weight. This makes many physicians reluctant to discuss weight control with their patients. But this problem, like any other, should be addressed. Patients need to hear the truth whether they like it or not.

Patients avoiding the truth are not a new problem. Alcoholics don't like to be told to stop drinking. Cigarette smokers don't like to be told to quit smoking. And diabetics don't like to be told that diet is a matter of life and death.

Many patients, left unchecked, develop weight gain insidiously. They don't notice that they are getting fat. Five pounds a year is less than a half a pound a month. But in 20 years, that's 100 pounds. Once a person is 100 pounds overweight, exercise is replaced by a sedentary lifestyle. Now somebody's gaining 10 pounds a year. It adds up quicker than you think.

All my patients at Aynor Family Practice were routinely weighed. Patients with any type of weight problem could expect to hear my concerns.

I would have been a lot more popular with some of my patients if I had bitten my tongue. My decision not to do so is based on my concern for patient health. I feel that physicians are obligated to identify and treat any preventable illness. This means inappropriate weight gain must be stopped. Obesity, when present, has be addressed.

Aynor Family Practice (AFP) scales could measure up to 1,000 pounds. These certified scales were extremely accurate and allowed us to effectively treat all overweight patients, including those with morbid obesity.

AFP's capacity to weigh patients is unusual. The ability to weigh overweight patients accurately is essential in any diet program.

STEP 2

Obesity is a big problem. Not everyone, that should, wants to address this problem. But ignoring the problem only makes the problem bigger. It might not be politically correct to lose weight by counting calories, but it's medically sound.

When I see obesity get bigger, I do make a big fuss — but I also try to help.

If losing weight was easy, there wouldn't be so many fat people. The correct diet for a diabetic is very simple...but hard work.

Lifelong diet is a lifestyle change. It is NOT a lifestyle change if it isn't everyday. Spend 10 minutes, EVERYDAY, reading this book. You can find something small you can do, but do it. Tomorrow, do something different.

Step 2

11. Eat Your Vegetables

The Number One cause of death in America is heart disease. The second leading cause of death is cancer. According to the *Journal of the American Cancer Society*, two-thirds of cancer deaths in the United States are self-inflicted. These deaths can be linked to tobacco use, poor diet, obesity, and the lack of exercise.

It's always been politically popular to blame the environment for cancer. The impact of the outside world on our health is a legitimate concern. Illegal dumps can contaminate water supply and cause cancer. As a general rule, these environmental problems account for a very small number of cancers: the worst environmental pollutants are the ones that we impose upon ourselves (e.g., smoking).

The coal mining industry is heavily criticized for exposing workers to conditions that can cause black lung. This disease, like emphysema, causes lung failure. Most people don't know that nine out of ten cases of black lung are the result of the combination of cigarette smoking **and** coal mining. Black lung is rare in employees who do not smoke. Ninety percent of black lung is self-inflicted, and not simply work-related.

The most common environmental pollutant is secondhand cigarette smoke. There is overwhelming evidence that in a closed environment, such as home or office, secondhand smoke for the nonsmoker is almost as bad as cigarette smoke is for the smoker. Sooner or later, this will need to be addressed politically.

People forget that tobacco products do not only cause lung cancer. They cause emphysema and heart disease. They increase the risk for many other cancers as well.

Alcohol consumption adds to cancer risk, especially for smokers. Breast cancer, colon cancer, bladder cancer, oral cancer and lung cancer are more common with the combined use of tobacco and alcohol. These "bad habits" contribute to oral cancer to such a degree that I have never seen oral cancer in a person who has never smoked or consumed alcohol.

Step 2

Much less publicized is the impact that poor diet, obesity, and the lack of exercise have on the risk for cancer. All three factors increase the probability of developing cancer (and heart disease!). These cancer risk factors are less known to most people.

For example, the relationship between the size of women and breast cancer has been well studied. Large women double their risk for breast cancer. Both men and women increase their risk for colon cancer as their weight increases.

Consumption of animal fat and the lack of fruits and vegetables in the diet seem to greatly increase the risk of several common cancers. Vegetable fat, monosaturated fat, and polysaturated fat have not demonstrated these problems. Large amounts of red meat, rather than fat, might be the true culprit. Colon cancer and prostate cancer seem to be the most affected. Ovarian and uterine cancer may be affected as well.

Eating fat and having a sedentary lifestyle increase the risk for obesity. Nevertheless, the issue seems to involve two separate risk factors. The first is weight and the second is diet.

An alternative to looking for harmful effects of diet is to find nutrients that reduce the risk for cancer. This idea is heavily promoted by herbal medicine advocates. The claim is that "natural" is *always* better and more is better still.

The most toxic known carcinogen (cancer-causing substance) known to man is a fungus spore produced by nature. Tobacco is a "natural" product that can be organically grown. Obviously more is not always better (e.g., fat).

Research has been successful in identifying a small number of specific beneficial vitamins and minerals. Folic acid supplements have clearly been shown to reduce birth defects, colon cancer and heart disease. Large amounts of selenium supplements were touted to reduce the risk of many cancers. Studies have shown that this is not true — with one exception. Prostate cancer seems to be less common with selenium supplements (but the definitive study is still pending). Excessive selenium is harmful.

Scientifically proven specific recommendations for diet and/or dietary supplements are difficult to find since research needed to fully understand these relationships take years to accomplish and are fraught with error. Furthermore, good diets high in fruits and vegetables contain large amounts of substances that have never been identified. Even products such as tobacco, which have been heavily researched, contain substances that we know nothing about. We do know that tar and nicotine are not the sole substances that cause cancer and/or heart disease.

Most dietary claims (including herbs and supplements) are not conclusively proven. Nevertheless, there is a clear need to increase Americans' consumption of fruit and vegetables. This has already been proven to prevent heart disease, the Number One cause of death in the U.S. Whether decreased fats or increased vegetables directly reduce the cancer rate is less clear. The data are overwhelming for the need to improve diet.

Many people on these diets (high fiber) also lose weight (less calories). Eating better, losing weight, and increasing exercise dramatically reduce your chances of developing many forms of cancer.

Many vitamins and minerals can be found in the balanced diet most Americans lack. Eating more fruit and vegetables means eating less meat and potatoes. *P. S.* Potatoes (most Americans call them French Fries) and corn are not vegetables; they are starches. (Most vegetables are green.) Cereals should be minimally refined and contain as much whole grain as possible. Avoid cereals (there are a lot of these) that have too much added sugar or caloric sweeteners (e.g., Raisin Bran)

Increased fiber may not help cancer but it definitely helps bowel movements and diabetes. Whole wheat bread has more fiber than white bread.

Thirty minutes of exercise a day dramatically improves weight control. Simply staying within the published weight guidelines is not sufficient to reduce cancer risk. The American Cancer Society goal is for adults to stay within 5 to 10 pounds of their weight at age 20. This guideline may seem extreme but it is the norm in Japan and in most parts of the world for adults.

Moderate alcohol consumption might help heart disease but it doesn't help cancer or beer bellies. I personally don't recommend alcohol consump-

Step 2

tion. My mom made me eat vegetables, not drink beer.

We are what we eat (or shall I say, overeat?). That's why many people in other countries live longer than we do. We just spend more on health care, usually trying to fix our mistakes. The biggest setback for health care looming in America is rising obesity. No vaccine, surgery, technology, chemotherapy, or pill can reverse this trend. Instead, we have to learn how to eat better.

My mom was right. Eat your vegetables. No more cookies; you can have a piece of fruit instead. No more soda, what's wrong with water? Quit lying around the house, go outside, and walk the dog.

I went to medical school so I could sound like my mom.

**If there is no need to change, why bother?
If there is a need to change, why stop?**

Step 2

12. Introduction: No Crap Diet for Diabetics

You probably wouldn't be reading this unless you, or someone you know, has been diagnosed with diabetes. Neglected diabetes makes people sick, so it is not a diagnosis that can simply be ignored. Patients with poorly controlled diabetes feel very badly and sometimes do worse.

In contrast, diabetics who maintain perfect blood glucose (sugar) control tend to do quite well. Most also feel well. The treatment for diabetes, correctly done, is very effective. Therefore, it is worth knowing how to treat diabetes. Any person, with this book and a doctor, can control diabetes.

If the treatment for diabetes were simple, every diabetic would have perfect blood glucose control. Most do not. For those who have started treating this disease, the task at hand does seem formidable. Many issues are complex and some are even controversial.

You want to begin by finding the most "bang for the buck."

It is hard to find the best solution if you do not understand the whole problem. Once you do understand the problem, you then also have to be willing to work on the solution. But then you have to know how. Only then can work began, one step at a time.

However, have you ever had a problem so big that you did not know where to begin? Have you ever been given directions so complicated that you did not know which way to turn? For many diabetics and their families, that is what diabetes has been — a big problem with complicated directions.

I have been a family practice doctor for more than fifteen years. Over the years, it has saddened me to see how confused patients are about diabetes and what they should do about it. Many want to do well, but do not know how or where to begin.

In order to achieve any goal, especially those hard to reach, someone needs to make it clear what these goals should be. Many patients and their families discover that modern medicine and scientists never seem to accomplish this. The language of science has many words that only a scientist really understands. "Experts" in the field of diabetes are still slugging it out on how

STEP 2

to treat this disease. It is not hard to understand why a lot of patients and their families are confused.

A doctor cannot do for you what you must do for yourself. Most people know this. But you cannot do well if it is not clear what needs to be done or where to start.

The "no crap" diet refers to both the need to eliminate junk food ("crap") from diet and the need to make an improved diet as straight forward as possible. The scientific babble commonly used in medical texts is "crap" most ordinary people do not need nor want to understand.

Much of the material in this book is simple. Some of it is very blunt. I do this to make important information and goals straightforward. The truth is not always what you want to learn. Nevertheless, it is what you **need** to learn. All "crap" stops here.

I have always received a lot of praise from my diabetic patients for being a good teacher. Some have also muttered that I am a good preacher. In any case, diabetics armed with better understanding make better patients. It is much easier for patients to decide how to control diabetes once the disease and treatment are clearly understood.

Some authors attempt to simplify problems by writing material at a third grade level. Doing so produces information designed for dummies. While the average diabetic is not college bound, the average patient is not stupid either. Anyone who can read or understand a newspaper should be able to follow my book.

This book is written for people who have common sense but are not necessarily interested in getting a degree in medicine. Everything is written to explain the "whys" and the "whats." Understanding the "whys" makes the "whats" a lot easier to remember and do. Easierrrrr, not necessarily easy.

When a lot needs to be done, a list of priorities needs to be created. When doing so, it is important to ignore information about diabetes or dieting that is trivial, not true, not healthy, too confusing, not important, or not helpful.Most reasonable people become confused by all the complicated con-

STEP 2

flicting advice the American Diabetic Association, dieticians, doctors, nurses, friends, relatives, books, articles etc., etc., can provide. A simple list of what to do that stands the test of time never seems to emerge. One year they tell you to do this and the next year they tell you to do something else.

At no time has the disease diabetes changed, but medical advice, goals, and priorities do so frequently. The harder some patients try to keep up and understand this disease, the less some do. It can be surprisingly hard to find clear goals to go by or which ones to begin with.

For other diabetics, the worst enemy they face is themselves. Even if it was easy to know everything that needs to be done to effectively control diabetes, most cannot simply do it. Part of who we are is the way we do things and old habits (including bad ones) are resistant to change. Reluctance to change "our ways" is a difficult obstacle for anyone to overcome.

Not surprisingly, every diabetic finds problems that seem difficult to solve. No one is perfect. This usually makes controlling diabetes, at some point, difficult to achieve. Solutions need to be found. If you are not part of the solution, you are part of the problem.

Diabetics cannot choose whether or not they have diabetes. Rather, diabetics can choose whether they will control diabetes, or let diabetes control them. It is well proven that diabetics who maintain normal blood glucose ("sugar control") can avoid complications caused by diabetes. They also feel so much better.

You can, with this book, recognize old habits that must be eliminated and new goals that have to be achieved. If you keep doing the same things, you will keep getting the same results. Therefore, "trying" doesn't count. Like it or not, disease can force us to face grim choices. Diabetes treatment is important. Die "trying" or do better with success are your best options.

The bad news is that there is no cure for diabetes. The good news is that diabetes is *one-hundred-percent* treatable... but it is a lifelong, lifestyle change. Some describe this treatment as a pain in the rear. I call it the "no-crap" diet for diabetics. You can call it what you want.

TEN STEPS To Control Diabetes requires: patience, perseverance,

Step 2

common sense, the three "Rs" (readin', ritin' and 'rithmetic), repetition to aid retention (in other words, two more "Rs"!), and a desire to stay alive.

If you feel the need to read the end of the book first, to see how it ends, don't bother. I will tell you now how it ends. The book ends as it begins: "you can't make chicken salad out of chicken crap." If you eat like an American, you will die like an American. The treatment of diabetes, unfortunately, demands dietary changes and not just medication.

It will take the entire book for you to understand what diabetes is, how diabetes needs to be treated, and what a diabetic must do. This book is designed to help the diabetic who does not want to be harmed by this disease.

TEN STEPS To Control Diabetes will show you the way, one small clear step at a time...

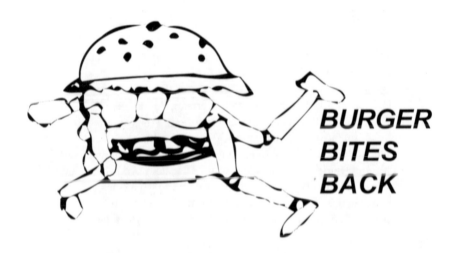

BURGER BITES BACK

Step 2

13. Fats, Fads, Facts, & Fiction

Often I am asked to give my opinion on the newest 'magical diet pills/ herbal remedies." I always say, "Cocaine use will also help you lose weight but that doesn't mean you should try it."

I generally have refused to recommend any diet pill, based on a long history of past failures. FDA (Federal Drug Agency) approval is no guarantee that a diet drug is safe.

Illness can cause appetite suppression followed by weight loss. Illnesses can be caused by medication. Be suspicious of any manufacturer's claim that their medication (including herbal) "only" suppresses appetite. It is not a sign of "wellness" to have no appetite.

Every year the New York Times Best Seller Book List includes at least one new diet book (or fad). Diet books are big business. So are diet pills. Dieting is a big business and it is very profitable.

Dieters want an easy and fast solution. The main theme used to attract buyers in the diet business is the promise that they don't have to count calories. In other words, it doesn't matter how much you eat, but rather, what you eat. They don't tell you that one can starve and become malnourished eating all the fruit one wants (e.g., the Hollywood diet). Fruit is water. A water diet is a starvation diet.

The second claim is usually some kind of pill or tonic that will cure obesity (e.g., Phen-Fen).

Baloney!

Diet programs sell the idea that there are "good calories" and "bad calories." Folks, a calorie is a calorie. A calorie is a measurement of energy (how much). Fuel (measured in calories) is used to make you go.

The body needs fuel to operate just like a gasoline engine needs gas. In people, the "engine" cannot ever stop. If it does, you die. The body converts food into fuel (glucose) which is measured in calories.

Unneeded fuel is stored as fat and muscle. Stored fuel can be used later for periods between meals. For immediate needs or when starving, muscle

Step 2

protein is converted into glucose. Fat is converted to glucose when slower and steadier amounts of glucose are needed.

Rapid weight loss will always result in loss of muscle mass (not fat). Because muscle is 90% water and water is heavy, dramatic weight loss can occur with starvation.

Losing large amounts of muscle mass is dangerous. Remember, the heart is a muscle. Many fad diets in the past have been taken off the market because of sudden death (heart attack).

LIFE IS NOT FAIR. Some folks can eat like a pig and be as skinny as a rail. Others look at food and gain weight. There is no question that people have different metabolisms and, therefore, different tendencies to gain weight.

How and why these differences occur, we do not fully understand.

In the past, attempts have been made to change metabolism in order to cause weight loss. Two old examples are amphetamines ("speed") and chemically-induced hyperthyroidism. Hyperthyroidism is a disease that can lead to many medical problems. "Speed," like cocaine, is not good for you. Occasionally, it can be fatal.

Most "fast and easy" weight loss plans are not lifelong solutions to a lifelong problem. The problem of obesity is very simple. If you take in more calories than you need, your body will store the extra calories as fat. If you want to lose weight, you will need to burn more calories than you take in. Lose weight slowly to "burn" fat.

It is medically impossible to lose more than one to two pounds of fat per week. People wanting to lose twenty pounds are looking at ten weeks (or more) of dieting. To maintain weight loss, new diets have to be permanent. There can be no temporary change in eating habits for permanent weight control.

There are diet plans that I can partially recommend. Weight Watchers and TOPS teach participants to eat a balanced diet. These plans are inexpensive and teach eating habits that you can live with forever. Talk to your doctor about plans you might be considering.

Step 2

Patients, while dieting, complain bitterly of increased appetite (hunger). Current suppressants (diet pills) are not without risks. The recall of Redux shows this to be true.

Hunger, to some degree, is learned behavior. Suppressing hunger requires behavioral changes. For example, patients who eat more when upset need to find other ways to relieve tension. Social activities, such as a date, need to be planned without eating.

How you perceive (see) things can be learned. Diets viewed as "punishments" will fail. Attitude can become very important. Can you enjoy dieting? Yes — with the right attitude.

One way to create some sense of stomach fullness is to eat a lot of low calorie, high fiber foods. A large pickle has 6 calories. A Big Mac and soda has 500 calories. 83 large pickles (500 calories) will kill anyone's appetite. Many could feel full with just 4 large pickles (which is only twenty-four calories). This is why an effective, but safe, weight loss program recommends foods low in calories and high in fiber. Be full — not fat.

One final myth: a low-fat gram diet will guarantee weight loss — *NOT TRUE*! If you drink orange juice (0 fat grams) all day, you will gain weight. What and how much you eat or drink *does* matter.

There are many low-fat items (both food and drink) with a lot of calories. Some labels heavily advertise their low-fat content. These items can still be full of sugar (i.e. table sugar). Sugar has no fat grams. Sugar does have a lot of calories. Excessive calories consumed are then converted to fat. Low-fat items can still be fattening. Count calories, not just fat grams.

Surgery is sometimes offered to treat severe obesity. Complications can be life threatening and/or disabling. These patients, even after surgery, are still required to diet. No one should undergo these procedures with the idea that dieting (a good diet) is unnecessary. However, for some people, surgery may be an answer. Time can only tell and you can't turn time back.

The other way to help lose weight is to burn more fuel. Caloric dietary restrictions can be less severe if you exercise. However, your feet cannot outrun your hands (you still must diet). Proper eating and exercise is the safe

Step 2

and best way to lose weight (as fat). Counting calories is necessary when trying to lose weight effectively and permanently.

There is no medicine that can change simple facts. You are what you eat. Some people have to work a lot harder to maintain ideal body weight.

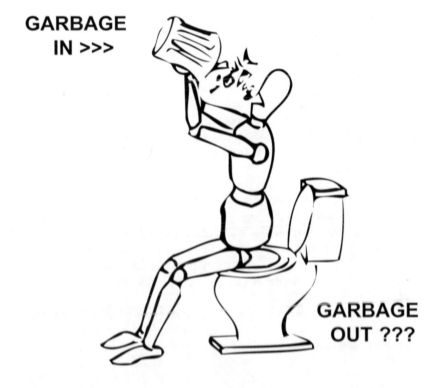

GARBAGE
IN >>>

GARBAGE
OUT ???

Step 2

14. The Battle of the Bulge

People don't always do things for the same reason. People eat for different reasons. Wrestlers eat to gain weight; others want to lose it.

Diet pills and surgery are not usually the solution for weight loss. Some of these strategies are designed to burn or waste calories. Many diseases do this same thing. If staying alive were not important, diet pills and surgery would be used more often.

Most diet pills are designed with the idea that hunger is the underlying cause of obesity. People are not that simple. People don't just eat because they are hungry.

If obesity were merely caused by excessive hunger, diet pills could be found that almost always work. They don't.

We don't eat simply for good nutrition. We are taught to relax and enjoy food. Eating is associated with pleasure. Food is usually selected for taste and not for its nutritional value. Taste is learned behavior.

Social gathering places, such as restaurants, tend to have food high in fat and sugar because that's what people like to buy and eat. Nutritious diets are not popular with many social activities of daily life (e.g., movies, etc.). "Diet" for the purpose of good nutrition (e.g., to lose weight) easily becomes a four-letter word.

We stop working to eat. If we only eat when we are relaxed, we learn to associate relaxation with eating. In time, for some, this association reverses. Relaxation becomes eating, i.e. in order to relax, I must eat.

Many studies show that some obese people struggle to lose weight because they eat to relax and not because they are hungry. People frustrated with obesity eat even more to calm themselves. This becomes a terrible and vicious cycle. "Diet" becomes a four-letter word that stimulates even more eating.

Many Americans are prejudiced against obese people. Studies show that obese people are viewed as stupid and lazy. A very competent, pleasant, and obese waitress will get smaller tips than a pretty, incompetent slim blonde.

Step 2

Obese people are less likely to be hired or promoted.

Contrary to these prejudices, obesity is not scientifically associated with stupidity. Granted, it is stupid to eat to relax and to try to overcome frustration about obesity with food. But it is also stupid to smoke, drink, and drive too fast. We are all stupid in some areas. Obese people are not any worse in this regard.

Contrary to common belief, obesity is also not scientifically associated with laziness. Studies show that obese people tend to be less active but this is not the same as lazy. Obese people tend to find ways to be more efficient so less energy is expended when working. Recreational activities tend to be sedentary. However, their willingness to initiate and complete work tasks is as good as anyone else's.

In fact, mild obesity is associated with increased work productivity. This is probably because obese people have to prove themselves more than others to keep a job, get a raise, etc.

The kind of food we like is taught to us by the people who raise us and by advertisers. We are taught that we should socialize while eating. Much of eating is therefore learned behavior. For all of us, it's very hard to unlearn what we frequently do as habit. We are particularly blind to our own bad habits. For those who need to change their diet, dieting is very difficult. "Diet" easily becomes a four-letter word.

Nasty comments are usually directed at people we don't like. We say things we know will offend these people. For the obese, "fat" is a popularly used insult.

Sports are usually played in public. In America, winning is considered to be very important (for some, it is everything). One strategy used to win is to insult your opponent.

If I learn that I look stupid while running, I tend not to run. America teaches obese people not to exercise. It is very common for perfect strangers to make nasty comments regarding "fat" when obese people are exercising or playing sports.

Finally, some people can eat a ton of food, not do a thing (lazy), and

Step 2

stay skinny. Contrary to popular belief, not all obese people eat "like a pig" at the dinner table. For many, decreased activity and efficient metabolism of food result in obesity.

In fact, some people need to eat much less food than others. This ability is lifesaving during famine but makes obesity much more likely when food is plentiful.

When I was young, I ate like a "pig," but I never became obese. For breakfast, I could eat a dozen eggs. At lunch, I could eat five Big Macs, large fries and a milk shake. Supper could easily be a one-pound package of spaghetti. Of course, I added a pound of hamburger to the spaghetti sauce, too.

Don't ask me where it all went. Thank God I was never in a concentration camp; I would have been the first one there to starve to death. Obviously my metabolism is considerably different from some who are obese.

Obesity is no longer a laughing matter. Obesity will surpass all other bad habits, such as smoking, as a public health problem.

Only recently have I picked up a few extra pounds. But I am not the only one. In America, we are literally eating ourselves to death, while many other parts of the world are starving to death. America is becoming fatter and obesity is rapidly becoming the Number One health problem for this country.

In 1944-45 (December-January), the Battle of the Ardennes, also known as the Battle of the Bulge, was won by the Americans. Today, we face a new "Battle of the Bulge" and we are losing the "battle" and not the weight.

Remember the commanding officer's gritty response — "Nuts" — when facing possible defeat. Courage and determination are critical ingredients for important battles to be won. However, the Battle of the Ardennes was not won solely by the men trapped in Bastogne. It was also won with help from the Allies (General Patton's troops along with the Air Force).

Obese people cannot seek refuge through pills or surgery. They need to unlearn bad behavior to lose weight. Attitudes must change about "diet" and exercise. Change cannot be temporary. It must be permanent.

But the Battle of the Bulge cannot be won alone. Everyone has a

Step 2

responsibility to improve the climate for people to eat and exercise properly. What are we feeding our children and our guests? Children need to learn good eating habits by example. Changes are needed in the way we socialize and celebrate holidays. Exercise is very boring for most people to do alone. Who's going to make the effort to exercise with someone else? Obese people are as normal as anyone else. The Battle of the Bulge cannot be won alone. Dieting is especially hard when you are surrounded by the enemy (Americans who eat like Americans).

Besides resolve, getting help from others is a very good idea for successful weight loss. Support Groups, such as Weight Watchers, TOPS, and exercise classes are extremely important allies for victory. Spouses, friends, and family should also be great allies. It is not a sign of weakness to depend on others for help.

No valor was lost when the men trapped in Bastogne were rescued by other American troops. But the determination ("Nuts") has to be there as well.

The first STEP to staying alive is to stop killing yourself with bad food.

Step 2

15. Why Eat and Drink?

Americans do like to eat and drink. More than half are overweight. That makes overweight "normal" in the USA. We are now the fattest country in the world.

A hundred years ago, Coke and Pepsi didn't exist. Neither did fast food. Currently, America drinks twice as much soda than milk. We spend more on alcohol than on milk or juices.

There is no question that American businesses would not advertise if it wasn't effective. America spends more on beverage advertising than on all education (including college) combined. Look whose logo is on your local high school signs. We consume more pounds of sugar than either beef or chicken. The effect mass media advertising has on American culture is quite evident. The result is a health care disaster.

When a human being becomes part of society, he/she learns from other people about all aspects of daily living. This includes eating and drinking. In this country, few Americans are Native Americans. We are all immigrants from other nations. Many past traditions and diets from these other countries have disappeared as our ancestors became "Americanized." Even Native Americans have become "Americanized." Recent immigrants tend to rapidly change the way they eat, too.

The forces that make so many people eat like "Americans" are very strong (whatever they may be).

We are what we eat (and drink). What America eats and how much we eat is not good. In spite of the fact that America spends more on health care than any other country, there are many nations whose citizens live longer than we do. Worse yet, many are countries (e.g., Europe) from which we immigrated. We may have their genes but not their diet.

Any developing country that adopts American's dietary habits sees a dramatic rise in diseases (e.g., diabetes) common in America. Eat like an American, die like an American.

America eats too much sugar, fat and meat. At least half of all cancers in America are diet-related. A high protein diet makes kidney stones more likely. We pass more kidney stones than any other country in the world. Our diets usually lack fiber (fruit, vegetables, and high fiber breads). This causes constipation. The U.S. buys more laxatives than the whole world combined. (Some things just aren't coming out right.)

Both the number of Americans who are overweight, and the rate at which this is occurring, are rapidly increasing. This problem goes hand-in-hand with diabetes (we're #1 there, too).

Whatever the reasons that Americans eat (quantity and quality), the concern about health is low on the list.

Even though the majority of Americans are overweight, the majority don't want to be. If it were easy to lose weight, there would be a lot fewer overweight people. The failure for most Americans to control weight is a reflection of how difficult it is to change eating habits. Again, whatever forces there are that influence our decisions about food and drink, they are very strong.

Members of any society tend to resist ending lifelong habits (no matter how desperately change is needed). Sooner or later, dieters forget how badly most Americans eat. Instead they continue to yearn for traditions as "American as apple pie." The hatred for dietary change and our love for "apple pie" are what makes most diet programs tiptoe around the need to abandon old eating habits.

For example, the American Diabetic Association (ADA) literature on the diabetic diet reassures American diabetics by stating "diabetes doesn't change the kinds of foods you eat." This is true — "diabetes doesn't" but new diabetics need to. One reason that diabetes is so common is because most diabetics have eaten like "normal" Americans. The truth is that most American diabetics must dramatically **change** the way they eat.

A concerned diabetic's primary purpose for eating is to maintain blood glucose (sugar) control and good health. It's not normal for most Americans to eat a nutritious diet in moderation or to eat small meals frequently. A healthy new diet for a diabetic will certainly contradict many American tradi-

Step 2

tions, including "apple pie."

Clearly most Americans choose food for other reasons (e.g., because it tastes good, etc.). A diabetic can tell you that trying to stay on a healthy diet can make you feel like a social outcast. There are very strong social pressures in America (e.g., Thanksgiving) that make a healthy diet very hard to maintain. Most obese dieters fail. A million Americans lose weight every year. A thousand keep it off.

Attitudes that resist needed change include: "I want to eat like every one else;" "they should make a diet pill so I can eat any way I want;" "it's unfair that I have this illness" (e.g., diabetes, obesity, etc.) and "diet is another form of punishment;" "I'll just die if I don't eat something that simply tastes good" (i.e. not necessarily good for you); "I just want to relax and have fun eating;" "I hate having to figure out how to eat healthier in contrast to everyone else;" and "I can't do this forever so I plan to stop dieting once I achieve my goal."

If a person is to be successful in dieting, one has to recognize that most people's reasons for eating are bad. Why you eat can affect what you eat. You can choose to either "eat to live" or "live to eat." Do you eat because it tastes good or do you eat because it's good for you? There is a difference.

It helps to develop a real hatred for how America eats. The American diet is killing you, your friends, and your family. If you eat like a normal American, you will probably suffer and die like one.

Whose funeral do you want to go to — yours or theirs? Food and drink is not worth dying for. From a health care point of view, it's stupid to eat like a "normal" American. America has a big need for a new diet; it just hasn't started yet. But this should not prevent **you** from changing **your** diet.

You can be smarter than the rest of the country. If you have a brain, why not use it before you put something in your mouth?

It is very important to remember that for whatever reasons America eats, it's not because Americans are trying to stay alive and well.

Step 2

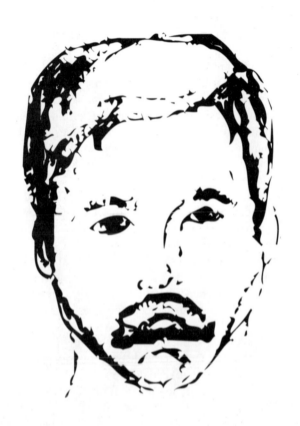

You feel as good as you eat

16. WHY YOU EAT AFFECTS WHAT YOU EAT

In poor countries, many people starve to death. In America, we eat ourselves to death. A diet can only help you if it is "good for you" and "it is for life."

Attitude and feelings are not the same. You control attitude but not your feelings. Hunger is a feeling that you cannot control. What you can control is your behavior to satisfy your hunger.

Hunger creates a desire to eat but attitude determines what you put in your mouth. People have many choices. Two examples include a diet pill that suppresses hunger or eating food until you are full. Many people who eat and drink are not hungry. There are many reasons a person would do this. For example, "It tastes good."

Food and water are the building blocks of life. (Our bodies are about 90% water.) All life depends upon food. Ideally we would never eat anything that is "bad" for us (toxic). However, human "intelligence" seems to choose food and drink for reasons other than nutrition.

Fortunately, most dietary errors are eliminated at the other end. Occasionally, they come back up. The kidney can also "void" mistakes.

We are what we eat when we don't eliminate it. Our mistakes add up. The increasing accumulation of toxic dietary mistakes eventually causes disease.

Medication is the most potent example of how food and drink can affect our health (and how we feel). It should be no surprise that large amounts of food or drink (albeit less potent) can do the same.

Disease lowers our ability to tolerate further dietary errors. In turn, dietary errors (a toxic burden) cause disease. This is a vicious cycle. While damage done cannot always be eliminated, tomorrow's health can still be improved by what you eat today.

The sole purpose of a healthy diet is to provide nutrients while minimizing the toxic burden of any dietary mistakes.

Stool and urine are things our body needs to eliminate. One man's

STEP 2

trash is another's treasure. (It's still trash for the first man.) Stool and urine provide needed nutrients (fertilizer) for plants. But for us, it's "crap" that needs to be eliminated.

Eating things that are not nutritious and/or are toxic needs to be eliminated from diet. If it's bad for us at one end, it will be bad for us at the other end, too.

The worst dietary mistake for an alcoholic is alcohol. The best treatment is **NO** alcohol. The worst thing for a drug addict is drugs. The best treatment is **NO** drugs. If your diet has a problem with a "sweet tooth," your solution is **NO** sweets (no sugar and no artificial sweeteners).

If the problem with the American diet is all the "crap" we eat (excessive fat, meat, and sugar with not enough fiber), the best treatment is **NO** "crap." Eat a potato, not a potato chip; eat a piece of fruit, not a piece of fruit pie; drink water, not sodas; etc..

Americans trying to "diet" complain that they are "just dying" (e.g., tastes s-o-o-o-o good) to keep eating or drinking their favorite kinds of "crap" (e.g., potato chip, pie, soda, etc.). Little do they realize, literally, how close they are to the truth. Are you dying to eat "crap" that needs to be eliminated from your diet? If you are, you are not alone. There do seem to be many Americans who only live to eat. These people don't seem to have much of a life and it will probably get even smaller.

Why we eat affects what we eat. If you want to stay healthy and live longer, the right diet is food that is "good for you." Most Americans choose to eat and drink a lot of "crap" for other reasons (e.g., "it tastes good"). You can't continue to eat for stupid reasons and expect to maintain your health. You need to decide whether you "live to eat" or "eat to live." You cannot do both. (You cannot have your cake and eat it, too.)

Most people begin a new diet to lose weight. If you are overweight, you are eating more calories than you need. To lose weight you need to reduce the number of calories you eat and drink. Since a lot of the "crap" Americans eat and drink is high in calories (sugar and fat), losing weight means **NO** "crap."

Step 2

To determine the right amount of fuel that your body needs, you must count calories. You cannot judge food by its cover, you must look in a book (i.e. calorie counter) or read the label to see what's in it.

It only makes sense that in order to reduce the number of calories you put in your mouth, you need to know where they are coming from. Counting calories helps you to determine what and how much food you should eat or drink. Quality and quantity are key ingredients in a healthy diet.

Exercise can help you lose weight and improve health as well. Exercise is important, but your feet cannot outrun your hands. A good diet is still the cornerstone to building good health.

Use common sense. A pill (e.g., diet pill) cannot fix what you put in your mouth. Since you have a brain, why not use it before you eat or drink. Your attitude about eating requires these thoughts: why do I eat; do "I eat to live;" or do "I live to eat"? There is a difference.

Let "why" affect "what" you eat. Again, it simply requires that you give more thought to your diet. Think before you eat or drink. You can control "what" you eat and drink. Food and drink that are not nutritious should be avoided. You can't make chicken salad out of chicken "crap." "Crap" always needs to be eliminated. It takes a lifetime of bad eating to become overweight, diseased, etc. It takes the rest of your life eating right to try to stay alive. We are what we eat.

Times change from time to time; fools don't. If there is no need to change the way you eat, why bother? If there is a need, why stop? There is no such thing as a "temporary diet" if "it is for life."

From a health care point of view, it's plain stupid to eat like a "normal" American. Intelligent people know that "an ounce of prevention is worth a pound of cure."

No one denies that it's nice when food that is "good for you" tastes good as well. But choosing food without regard for nutrition (e.g., because "it tastes good") has certainly proven to be harmful in this country. The national data is overwhelming: it matters why you eat, what you eat, and how much you eat.

S-o-o-o, why do **you** eat...?

STEP 2

THE UNBALANCED AMERICAN DIET

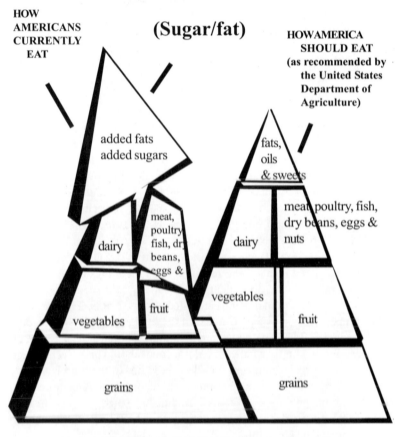

HOW AMERICANS CURRENTLY EAT

(Sugar/fat)

HOW AMERICA SHOULD EAT (as recommended by the United States Department of Agriculture)

added fats
added sugars

fats, oils & sweets

dairy

meat, poultry fish, dry beans, eggs &

meat poultry, fish, dry beans, eggs & nuts

dairy

vegetables

fruit

vegetables

fruit

grains

grains

Source: United States Department of Agriculture
Food Review 23, 3 (2000): 13, figure 3.

17. SIMPLY READ A FOOD LABEL

You can't judge food by its cover. You must read the label or look it up in a book (i.e. calorie counter). Food labels have become very complicated. They can be simplified (you'll see).

The first thing you should check is "serving size." Never assume the information on the label represents the entire contents of the package. Never assume that "serving sizes" are reasonable. The label will tell you how many servings there are in a package. If you are interested in comparing the label of one brand with another, make certain that your serving sizes are equal (comparable).

The next item of interest is calories. Everything (except water) has calories (it's not "if" but "how many"). It doesn't matter where the calories come from (whether it's fat, carbohydrates or protein). A calorie is a calorie. A calorie represents how much fuel there is in food or drink. You need energy to go. If you run out of "gas," you die. Excessive fuel is stored as fat in the body. If you want to lose weight, you need to determine where the excessive fuel is coming from. This is done by counting calories (not fat grams, "carbs," "points," exchanges, etc.).

The United States Department of Agriculture (USDA) recommends that you eat balanced meals. The recommended quantities of a variety of vitamins and minerals are dependent on how many calories a person eats. Many of these vitamins and minerals are listed on food labels. The quantities of these items are listed as a percentage of the total amount recommended. This is based on a specific calorie count mentioned somewhere on the label. (In no way does that imply what your calorie count should be.) Even though the USDA gives precise numbers for all of these items, the truth is that we really don't know what the precise numbers should be. USDA recommendations for vitamins and minerals are reasonable "educated guesses" of how much we need. Excessive amounts of some minerals and vitamins are harmful. Therefore, goals are helpful.

Precisely adding up vitamins and minerals is not helpful. So don't do it. There is no point in this kind of mathematical precision. If you eat a balanced meal, you will probably get all the vitamins and minerals you need. Food label percentages could help you learn which foods have what and how much, but you do not have to learn any of this. The USDA's "pyramid of food" is well-publicized and gives a general picture of what a balanced diet should consist of. That is good enough.

You can also take a once-per-day multivitamin to minimize any possibility that an essential vitamin is lacking in your diet. Remember, too much of anything can be bad. More is not always better. "Mega" vitamins are not risk-free.

Food labels do not merely list fat content. Fat is broken down into saturated fat, polyunsaturated fat, and mono-unsaturated fat. (Cholesterol, which is a fat, is listed as a separate item.) The problem with all fat is that many people eat too much of all kinds. Fat is high in calories and has no fiber. Eating excessive calories makes you fat. A low-fat diet means less calories from fat but will not exclude foods high in sugar and calories (so count calories). If you like to eat "carbs" or sweets, a low-fat diet can get you into a lot of trouble.

I do not see much purpose in counting fat grams or monitoring the percentage of "saturated" and "unsaturated" fats indicated by food labels. The "polys" and the "monos" interest me even less. If you are overweight or have had a heart attack, eat fewer calories. Any reduction in caloric intake tends to reduce all fat consumption (since fat is high in calories). Simply count calories.

Most Americans need to increase the amount of fiber they eat. If this is done, and total caloric intake is unchanged, the amount of fat per meal will automatically fall even more (Fat has no fiber.). Therefore, you can easily reduce excessive fat intake by decreasing or maintaining calories *while* you increase dietary fiber.

The total elimination of dietary fat is not healthy. Dietary fat is an essential ingredient to a balanced meal. (But only small amounts are needed.) The amount of fat you will need is naturally contained in some foods you should eat (e.g., fish). Avoid deliberately adding any fat to your diet (e.g., chips). Avoid eating fatty food you know as "junk" food ("crap").

Many patients have been told to "avoid cholesterol." Labels indicate cholesterol as a separate item. Some packages brag about their cholesterol content. None of this is very important with regards to blood cholesterol. For most people, the importance of *dietary* cholesterol on *blood* cholesterol is greatly exaggerated. Cholesterol is high in calories and has no fiber, so counting calorie/fiber will (again) address this concern. A low calorie, high fiber diet is a low cholesterol diet.

All labels list sodium. Sodium is "salt." It is an unavoidable compo-nent of food and is essential to life. There is no such thing as a diet without salt. While most Americans eat too much salt, for most, it is a harmless mistake. For no logical reason, a lot of processed high salt food (e.g., pizza, potato chips, etc.) are also high in calories. This, not salt, is the problem for most people. Excessive salt can be dangerous for patients with kidney or heart problems. Restricting salt intake is done by eliminating the use of a salt shaker (don't add salt) and by avoiding processed foods that are high in salt (e.g., sausage). For most Americans, salt restriction and the salt content of food is not a big concern.

Potassium is another kind of "salt." Patients with severe kidney prob-lems need to be attentive about this type of salt. For the rest of us, it's not something we need to read about on the label. If you are low in potassium, have your doctor prescribe a potassium supplement (no calories).

Food labels also indicate protein content. Meats, eggs, and dairy products are our greatest sources of protein (and usually a source of fat, as well). The food pyramid gives an approximate picture, calorie wise, of how much protein (and some fat, which is okay) you should eat in relation to everything else. Most Americans eat too much protein (and fat). Protein has no fiber but does have calories. Eating fiber in approximately the right ca-loric portions (e.g., food pyramid) eliminates the need to "protein count." A high protein diet is filling and low in calories but it is also constipating and a risk factor for "stones," heart disease, stroke, and/or cancer.

STEP 2

Eating more fiber without increasing calories reduces protein intake because protein has no fiber. I am not advocating an all fiber, no meat diet (e.g., vegetarian diet). A measured amount of protein (e.g., one egg, fish, dairy product, etc.) is part of a healthy balanced diet.

Carbohydrates are always listed on a food label. That's what "carbo" counters count. Bread, grain, fruit, vegetables, starch, and "sugar" are all carbohydrates. If food has calories and is not pure protein and/or fat, it must contain some carbohydrates. Plants store fuel as a carbohydrate. Blood glucose is a carbohydrate. If it's not greasy, oily, cheesy, milky, meaty, or nutty-it probably is a carbohydrate. "Sweets" are carbohydrates. Not all carbohydrates have dietary fiber but all dietary fiber has carbohydrates. If calories stay the same, but intake of dietary fiber goes up, then more food will be from carbohydrates that have fiber. So a low calorie, high fiber diet is a diet that has the correct amount of high fiber carbohydrates. Too much of anything is bad. In healthy diets, carbohydrates will provide the bulk of needed calories. The big base of the food pyramid (vegetables, fruit, bread, etc.) is made up of carbohydrates. Carbohydrates with fiber are a preferred choice, but not all carbohydrates selected will have fiber (which is okay for variety sake).

The most confusing aspect of food labels is "sugar." Most people think of table sugar (which is "sucrose") when "sugar" is mentioned. Sucrose (table sugar) is made from sugar cane. Sugar cane is a plant and plants store fuel as carbohydrates. Refined sucrose is a purified substance removed from sugar cane that is pure energy (fuel) and, therefore, high in calories. It also taste very sweet, which is why it is sought. This sweet carbohydrate is a simple "carb" molecule that has been named "sucrose." All fiber and other nutrients are removed when this carbohydrate is produced... then there is fructose, dextrose, and other "oses"...

Corn is a "starch." This carbohydrate can be refined to make "corn sweeteners," a popular sucrose substitute. Like sucrose, corn sweeteners are separated from fiber and other nutrients. Alcohol is another refined "sugar" or carbohydrate made from corn. Alcohol is not sweet, but like sucrose, is

Step 2

pure energy devoid of any fiber or nutrients.

Any refined sweetener with calories is a "sugar" (or carbohydrate) that is low in fiber and high in calories. Almost all foods contain some "sugar" (i.e. "carbs"). All "sugar" is not "bad." Fruit contains "sugar." Sugar (like salt) cannot be totally eliminated from a healthy diet. There cannot be a "no sugar" diet.

What does need to be eliminated is high calorie, no fiber (i.e. "crap"), plain table sugar (sucrose), other refined caloric sweeteners, and alcohol. More than 150 pounds (per year) of caloric sweeteners is added to American food and drink (e.g., sodas). That is a lot of "empty" calories. Most Americans are **not** deficient in calories. No one needs these kinds of carbohydrates.

Reducing calories and increasing dietary fiber helps avoid excessive refined "sugars" and alcohol. Refined sugar or alcohol is high in calories and low in fiber.

Whole fruit, like whole grain or vegetables, is a carbohydrate that has fiber. Whole fruit is not "pure energy." Whole fruit is nutritious and has fiber. Eating the right number of calories and as much fiber as possible allows whole fruit to be included as a healthy choice. Eat fruit, don't drink it. Juice is fruit without fiber and is high in "sugar," just like sodas with sucrose are.

What about red wine? It is not pure alcohol (so some nutrients managed to survive) but it is no diet drink. Wine is like juice, high in calories and low in fiber (like sodas). If you want to prevent heart disease, take a zero calorie cholesterol-lowering medication (less liver side-effects) with a low calorie, high fiber diet.

"Carbo" counting treats sucrose, alcohol, and whole fruit as the same...pretty sad idea unless you want to die drinking sweet beer. Quality counts, so count calories and fiber.

All the basic food groups are pictured on the USDA food pyramid. A healthy diet consists of eating a variety of food in moderation (correct calorie count) and in the right proportions (balanced with fiber). The greatest

Step 2

sources of fiber are located in the lower half (i.e. base) of the pyramid. S-o-o-o, the only numbers you probably need to read on the label are calories and fiber. At least two thirds of your calories should include fiber, preferably from whole grains, fruit, and vegetables (as close to the garden as possible).

Some final points: milk and water are the only two beverages you need (especially water). Milk is part of a meal (e.g., add to a high fiber cereal), not a thirst-quencher (skin milk has a lot of calories). Most Americans need to eat more fiber. **EAT** fruit, **NEVER** drink it. Your easiest source of fiber is high-fiber cereal and brown bread (but watch the calories). Eat more vegetables. Many people need to eat less red meat, cheese, or eggs and eat more fish. Too much fat, protein, or "sugar" is bad. Too many calories of anything makes you fat (gain weight).

When eating, counting calories is what counts. Then fill up on as much fiber as possible. Read the label for the numbers of these two items. When thirsty, drink water, period.

Is that simple enough?

**EAT A LITTLE OF A LOT,
RATHER THAN A LOT OF A LITTLE.**

---

18. Nearer the Needle, Further the Forest

Popular medical advice and opinion can have tremendous economic impact. When the American Heart Association recommended decreased egg consumption, a lot of family-owned egg farms went out of business. When increased dietary fiber was recommended, manufacturers started adding sawdust to food. When table sugar (sucrose) consumption became concerning, corn syrup and artificial sweeteners became a billion-dollar business.

It was hoped that labeling food products would help improve nutrition. Consumers with health concerns can now seek or avoid a variety of ingredients, such as cholesterol, fat, fiber, etc. One product can pit itself against another based on one or more ingredients. How this can be done depends on food labeling laws. The medical-legal definition of ingredients has become extremely controversial and complex.

A lot of the important science on nutrition started with agricultural research. But the nutrients being studied were those needed to improve production of agricultural products (e.g., better feed for cows).

In medicine, the concern is the nutrition for mankind. The concept of fiber came from agricultural research. The initial concept of fiber was very simple...fiber is the undigested remnants of plants (e.g., cow feed).

But different animals have different digestive systems. Cows digest plants/vegetables better than humans, so that the definition of fiber can be contingent on which animal is actually doing the eating. Even within the same species (e.g., animal), the amount of fiber found coming out at the other end can vary.

But food labeling laws require precise measurements.

Another definition for fiber is to establish a laboratory standard. You can mix some stomach acid with food in a test tube and declare the remnants as fiber. Unfortunately, some of these results may not resemble any result produced by man or cow (at the other end). Controversy can also develop on how much acid or food should be used. Laboratory standards can create a war over whose standards should be chosen.

STEP 2

A biochemist can step in and define fiber by chemical structure. Others will come forward and argue for different structures. When all is said and done, what is fiber can become a very complex question.

One way or the other, wheat usually is used to make bread. White flour is highly processed grain where most of the natural wheat fiber is removed, as well as the natural nutrients. If you keep wheat fiber, you make brown bread. If you make white flour, you remove wheat fiber.

The nutritional significance for fiber may not be the fiber itself, but where it came from. Fiber attached to wheat may not have the same nutritional impact as fiber found in sawdust. White flour mixed with sawdust can produce high-fiber bread just as whole grain wheat can produce high-fiber bread. Sawdust is an inexpensive source of fiber. But the quality of nutrition may not be the same.

Some consumer groups have protested that the addition of sawdust to improve fiber content of food should not be allowed, unless sawdust is listed as "sawdust." Manufacturers do not want to list sawdust as a source of fiber. Current law requires that total fiber content simply be listed. The sources of fiber does not have to be detailed (by definition, it comes out the other end undigested).

You might be curious to know how to detect the possibility that your high-fiber bread contains a lot of sawdust.

"Enriched" white flour means that some nutrients removed have been artificially reintroduced. And th-e-e-e-n fiber can to be reintroduced (added). When manufacturers want to increase fiber content of low-fiber white flour, sawdust is the cheapest additive.

It's important to understand that the precise ingredients of a high-fiber diet that make this diet healthier than a low-fiber one are not known. Obviously, older studies that reported huge health benefits from a high-fiber diet did not look at patients who were being fed high-fiber diets using fiber from sawdust. Since the true underlying reason why a high-fiber diet is healthier is not known, it would be wise to use the ingredients that we know work (which are whole-grains, whole wheat, etc.).

Step 2

Even if fiber itself has no nutritional value, it still has important dietary impact. Fiber has an important mechanical effect on the digestive system. By definition, the bulk that forms stool is fiber.

Without a bulking agent mixed with water, stools would become either very firm (constipation) or very poorly formed (diarrhea). Both conditions can affect the absorption of other nutrients so that stool consistency can affect overall well-being.

In a reasonably well-designed food label, fiber (simply defined as undigested food) is needed as a listed ingredient.

But when a group of lawyers and scientists with a variety of interests got together, finding an agreeable medical and legal definition of the word "fiber" was not so easy. Hairsplitting really starts when the definition of words affects someone's cash flow.

A *vague* definition of fiber opens the door for manufacturers to use any source of fiber, such as sawdust. A *strict* biochemical definition might have excluded fiber content of whole wheat which may have nutrients that prevent disease.

Looking at pine needles doesn't give the same picture as looking at the forest. The most compelling evidence about the value of a high fiber, low calorie diet is a view of the forest. But the best legal definition of fiber looks at pine needles. Neither view sees the same picture, but both views are looking at the same trees. Even today, issues about fiber remain controversial.

So in addition to looking at calories and fiber, it's probably also wise to look at the ingredients listed on a food label. Ingredients are listed in descending order. The largest fraction is listed first. Trivial ingredients are listed last.

Learn the names of common, sometimes controversial, ingredients. Choose ingredients as close to the garden as possible. When it comes to flour, look for whole grains. Avoid white flour, sucrose, caloric sweeteners and artificial sweeteners. If both flours are listed, see which one is listed first. Small amounts of added "crap" is sometimes unavoidable, but big "piles" are not.

Step 2

What bread is made of may be more important than most people realize. Looking only at calories/ fiber won't tell you that.

Over time, you will learn what all that crap listed really means.

YOU CAN ONLY FEEL AS GOOD AS YOU EAT.

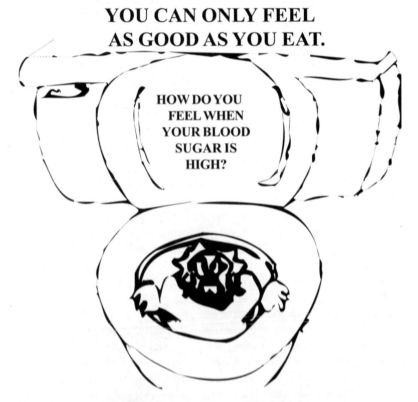

HOW DO YOU FEEL WHEN YOUR BLOOD SUGAR IS HIGH?

WHAT YOUR BODY DOESN'T NEED SHOULD BE ELIMINATED. YOU ARE WHAT YOU EAT WHEN YOU CAN'T.

Step 2

19. Remember Me, Type 1?

Obesity is a common problem for Type 2 diabetics. In contrast, it is **not** usually a problem for Type 1 diabetics. Ninety to ninety-five percent of diabetics are Type 2. However, not all Type 2 diabetics are overweight.

What are the dietary goals for thin diabetics (Type 1 or 2)? Not too different from fat ones. Six small nutritious meals per day, eat as much fiber as possible, count calories because calories count, and eat to live rather than live to eat.

The big difference in diet between skinny diabetics and fat ones is that obese diabetics need to lose weight. Overweight diabetics carefully count calories to try to avoid any excessive calories. Skinny diabetics count calories to be sure they have enough calories to avoid any hypoglycemia.

It is important to remember that Type 1 diabetics and Type 2 diabetics suffer from two different diseases. Different diseases with different problems. Obviously, they have different issues too.

The biggest lifelong issue for many Type 1 diabetics is hypoglycemia ("low sugar"). The larger issue for Type 2 is hyperglycemia ("high sugar")...

Many Type 1 diabetics develop their disease in their youth. They are thin and vulnerable to low sugar. Eating extra seems harmless. Eating more often, prudent.

Many Type 2 diabetics struggle with obesity for years before diabetes shows its ugly head. Initially, low sugar is rare. Eating more often is unappealing and eating too much of the wrong things is a lifelong battle.

The latest fad is "carbo" counting. "Experts" believe this is the most important factor to consider when deciding insulin dosage, an issue that is very important to brittle Type 1 diabetics. I do not have enough expertise or experience with Type 1 diabetics to agree or disagree. I **do** know that a high fiber diet will help prevent hypoglycemia and hyperglycemia. A high fiber diet makes blood glucose control less "brittle."

Type 2 diabetics hope a low-carb diet (e.g., Aktin's diet) is an easy way to lose weight. Easy? Maybe. Healthy? Doubtful.

Step 2

A high fiber diet is a high "carbo" diet, but fiber counts too.

It is much easier for a Type 1 diabetic to actually pass out from severe hypoglycemia than a type 2 (but some type 2 patients are pretty good at this too). For these patients, preventing hypoglycemia is definitely a more lifelong concern than either hyperglycemia or weight control.

(Good practical reading for the treatment of hypoglycemia is a book by two Type 1 diabetics: T. A. Lincoln and J. A. Eaddy, both physicians. It's called *Beating the blood sugar blues: proven methods for controlling hypoglycemia,* copyrighted 2001, Publisher ADA.)

For Type 1 diabetics, might "carbo" counting be better when one actually has low "sugar"? I doubt it. A high fiber diet has been proven to be the best solution for preventing this dangerous problem. When treating severe hypoglycemia, you are looking for low fiber "carbs." Once again, fiber cannot be ignored.

Most diabetics are Type 2. Their biggest lifelong issue is commonly obesity. This is usually caused by a high calorie, low fiber diet. To fix that problem, both calories and fiber need to be counted and changed. Counting just "carbos" makes no sense. Just as counting only fat grams makes no sense. Nor does counting primarily protein. So just count calories and fiber... (just that simple!).

If a dieter has a sweet tooth, they are more willing to reduce fat grams than carbs. Sugar lovers counting fat grams can still have and eat their cake (if it is fat-free). If you are overweight, the problem is in what you like to eat and not what you are not eating. Obviously, a low fat, high sugar diet is not a healthy choice if 90% of the calories are from cake. But that is what a sweet tooth counting fat grams can achieve.

One reason weight-losing diets fail is that obese patients can pick from many diets the "diet" they hate the least and avoid one they need the most. It is only human to hate losing the things you love.

The ADA takes the position that table sugar (sucrose) has the same impact as an equivalent amount (calorie-wise) of starch (e.g., potato) on blood sugar. I do not believe many Type 1 diabetics would choose a potato over sugar if severely hypoglycemic. Drinking sugar (e.g., soda) is not the same as sucking, eating, or drinking a potato. However, even if this were possible, the long term health consequences of eating a pound of sugar versus a pound of potatoes, every three days, is clearly not the same.

A high calorie, low fiber diet (e.g., the normal American diet) is the greatest predictor for the tendency of a nation's population to develop Type 2 diabetes, but not Type 1. A diet high in sugar is a high calorie, low fiber diet. A baked potato diet is not. But french fries are. How and what we eat has tremendous affect on what diseases we see.

A diabetic addicted to sweets might find it easier to stop eating too many potatoes rather than too many sweets.

Counting "carbs" ignores these important dietary issues.

It has been proven that a low calorie, high fiber diet can prevent Type 2 diabetes. No good proof exists for "carbo" counting.

A low calorie, high fiber diet has been proven to prevent heart attack and strokes. No such proof exists for "carbo" counting. Type 1 diabetics can suffer from heart disease just like Type 2 patients. Why then, would these diabetics want to ignore dietary fiber?

It remains to be proven if these two different types of diabetics really need to be on the same diet, but I will still put my money on a high fiber diet for both. Calories? That has to be counted...and that will differ.

I have been asked many times about "carbo" counting. I have no need, therefore no interest, in counting anything more than calories and fiber.

EAT LESS
BUT
MORE OFTEN

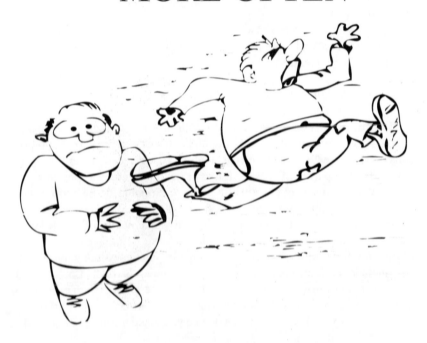

SO YOU WON'T RUN OUT OF GAS
If you want to have normal blood glucose control,
six small meals per day is not negotiable

20. *STEP 2* FOR CONTROL OF DIABETES

The first step to staying alive is to stop killing yourself with bad food. You have two choices. Live to eat or Eat to live. Your diabetes can control you or you can control your diabetes. Life is worth dieting for. Today is the second step towards *your control* of diabetes.

Goals for STEP 2:
Everything you needed to know previously was in Step 1. Know (don't just read) all the chapters before this chapter, Step 2. This second step has two parts: Quality & Quantity.

Improving the Quality of Food Consumed. Be sure to read: *16. Why You Eat Affects What You Eat* and *17. Simply Read a Food Label*.
A. Eat more fiber (e.g., eat fruit, don't drink it). Eat high-fiber cereals (e.g., no grits or cream of wheat). Eat high-fiber brown bread (e.g., no biscuits or white bread). Eat more vegetables (e.g., less meat). Over time, you will find more sources of "fiber." Eat as close to the garden as possible.
B. Use common sense; cut out the "crap." No junk food, i.e. **no** sodas, cakes, cookies, chips, fast-food, pizza, fried or greasy food, candy, ice cream, sugar (including sweet tea and Kool-Aid), dairy creamer in coffee, etc., etc., etc.). This will also help you reduce "calories."
C. Start a "food diary." Write down anything that goes into your mouth. This includes all food and drink. The only exception is water. Look at food labels to note calories and fiber for items that are packaged. Try to keep good records so your doctor can see what you're eating on your next office visit. This diary will help you to the degree you make it work (by doing it!).

Improving the Quantity of Food Consumed — Eat Less, But More Often. Eat six times per day. "Eat less, but more often." If you are overweight, eat a *lot* less, but *still* more often. If you are overweight, you should understand:

STEP 2

10. Why the Big Fuss, and *11. Eat Your Vegetables;*
13. Fats, Fads, Facts, & Fiction and *14. The Battle of the Bulge.*

Questions commonly asked by patients:

What is "crap" ????? Food that is not nutritious, and for a diabetic, harmful (e.g., candy, pure sugar ...). Food that has had fiber removed and calories added when compared to its "natural" state (e.g., potato chips from potato, juice from fruit ...). Anything high in fat (e.g., fried food instead of boiled, ice cream ...). Anything high in "calories" (e.g., pizza).

I thought juice was good for you? That's what advertisers want you to believe. Diabetics need fiber. You make juice by removing fiber. Therefore, fruit is better. How many oranges does it take to make one glass of orange juice? LOTS! You would never eat that many oranges at one time. In other words, you would never consume that many calories eating fruit (just drinking it). Reread your chapters from Step 1 if you do not understand this answer to this question.

Why can I eat better (dieting) but still gain weight? Weight gain can be a sign that your high blood glucose is lower because of improved diet. As blood sugar falls, a person can no longer urinate extra sugar (calories) that leaks into the bladder when blood glucose is too high. In other words, extra calories eaten can no longer simply go "down the toilet." Instead, it has to be stored as fat. Even though some diabetics are eating less calories than before, their "diet" is only good enough to improve blood sugar (glucose). Weight control will require further improvement in diet (even less calories). For these diabetics, if weight gain is not stopped, blood glucose (sugar) will soon rise again (so will insulin resistance).

Why not keep my sugar "high" so I can lose weight easily? Because "high" glucose (uncontrolled diabetes) will make you very sick and eventually kill you (much sooner than you want). Dead people lose weight too. **Both** weight **and** glucose need to be controlled.

Why can't I skip meals to lose weight? Because diabetics get "low sugar" (low blood glucose) as well as "high sugar." If you starve too much, you can die from "low sugar."

Why don't other diabetics eat that way — "more often, but less" ("it makes me hungrier to eat more often"), ("I don't have time"), ("I've always skipped breakfast"), ("I can't eat when I'm working"), (etc., etc. ...). Whether a diabetic realizes it or not, diabetes can kill. Some don't do what needs to be done. Diabetics who refuse to diet properly will probably die from diabetes. You really have to do this: eat less, but more often (i.e. control weight and blood sugar). Reread your chapters from Step 1 if you don't understand. *This is hard! Can you help me?* Sure. Imagine that you eat three reasonable low**er** calorie, high**er** fiber meals per day — breakfast, lunch, and dinner. Adjust each meal to be about the same number of calories. Dinner should no longer be the "big meal of the day." Divide each meal in half. Store half for later. Eat each half two to three hours apart. Now you have six small meals per day (last one at bedtime), **and** you don't have to prepare any more meals than normal (3). You don't use "crappy" snacks between meals. It is important to remember that you do not have to prepare more meals, you just have to use more food storage "baggies."

What if I've never eaten three meals a day (breakfast, lunch, dinner)? Okay, try it this way. Imagine all the food you normally eat in one day (24 hours). Put it all out on a table at one time. Eliminate the "crap" and improve the quality. If you are overweight, remove some more food. Now take what's left and divide it into six small piles (meals). You don't necessarily have to divide a single food item. You can eat the meat separately from the potato. There's not much extra work with this arrangement. Just better meal planning (and more food baggies).

What does "low sugar" (the medical word is hypoglycemia) feel like? It varies. Usually, you rapidly don't feel well. You might feel drunk, lightheaded, or pass out. You can feel any of the following: weak, sweaty, nervous, clammy, or unusually hungry. Check your sugar if you think you are hypoglycemic. Once confirmed, you now know what low sugar feels like for you. Be sure to let your doctor know you're having this problem, but first eat something quickly! Hypoglycemia is very dangerous. Don't skip meals !!!!

Questions your doctor might ask you:

Do you know all your medication bottles?
Do you still want to live — in other words, are you trying to change your diet?
Did you write down everything that went into your mouth (bring your food diary)?
Do you have any questions, concerns, or problems?

Food Guide Pyramid
A Guide to Daily Food Choices

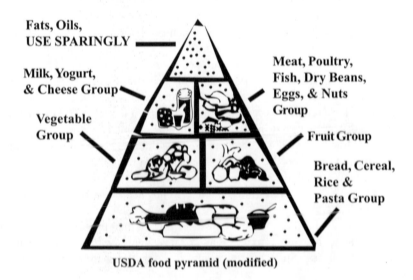

USDA food pyramid (modified)

STEP 3

21. THE MEANS AND THE GOAL

After many months of regular exercise and proper diet (i.e. the means), most people feel better (the goal). Patients on medications usually find it necessary to reduce or eliminate dosages. Arthritis, hypertension, and diabetes seem to particularly benefit. Sleep and energy usually improve. Depression can get better. Even the risk of cancer goes down.

Correct calorie consumption with increased fiber content can result in permanent weight loss without excessive hunger. This success is usually only possible after many lessons are learned and changes are accepted.

Correct calorie intake has a wide range. The more difficulty an individual has had with obesity, the more strictly enforced proper caloric intake must be maintained. Correct caloric intake is never negotiable. The correct count must be accepted if weight loss is to be achieved and maintained.

Even rare violations of dieting have devastating effects on weight control. It takes months or years to build a house from scratch but a house can be burned down in a matter of minutes. Dieting can take months or years to achieve goals, but weight gain can be achieved in days. One birthday cake can wipe out a week's worth of dieting. (Who said life was fair?)

Overweight Americans cannot eat like other Americans. One reason that more than half of the people in the USA are overweight is because Americans eat too much fat and sugar. Most Americans easily exceed their required caloric intake. Successful dieters learn not to eat like "Americans." Old favorites (food or drink items) are forever avoided.

Most obese calorie counters are astounded over the number of calories that are really needed to achieve and maintain weight control. Cutting caloric intake in half does not mean body weight will be halved. Some dieters need to cut calories even more than half to just achieve a 10% reduction in weight.

Foods that are forever removed from the menu needed for weight control range from juices to ice creams. These items, by their nature, cannot be low in calories. Sugar content and/or fat content demand that these items

STEP 3

not be consumed. No if's, and's, or but's.

What is there about "no" that cannot be understood? Is it the "n" or the "o"? "No juices" means *nooooo* juices. Failure to lose weight is failure to accept and maintain needed dietary changes — **absolutely!** Indeed, no one ever dies from not drinking sweetened drinks even though some people believe they just can't live without it. Believing one will die without bad things in his or her diet results in failure to improve diet.

It's very easy to get too many calories from food (e.g., cakes) or drinks (e.g., sodas, sweet tea, etc.) that are not filling but tastes good. This kind of "crap" is high in calories and low in fiber. A good diet is low in calories and high in fiber. It cannot be emphasized enough—you cannot make chicken salad out of chicken crap. No matter how much a dieter loves some food and drinks, American dietary "crap" needs to be eliminated (permanently).

Changing is more painful than the change itself. High-salt consumers, once accustomed to low-salt diets, will rarely resume eating excessive salt again. It tastes too salty if old quantities of salt are reintroduced. It's the getting there that's hard.

Dieting is the same. Losing items is worse than items lost and forgotten. The further along changes have been accomplished, the less the old ways are missed.

Practice makes perfect. Repetitive rituals, such as calorie counting, become easier after many months of practice. In fact, one can get quite good at it and what was a chore becomes a breeze.

Calorie counters discover a lot of old myths. For example, many are surprised that the caloric difference between whole milk and skim milk is rather small. Even skim milk has more calories than most sodas. Similar products can have tremendous differences in calorie content. Different brands of spaghetti sauce can differ by more than 200 calories (8 oz.).

Calorie counters learn that calories add up quickly. Eating an avoidable (and extra) 200 calories can make the difference between weight loss and weight gain. Caloric differences of 200 calories can represent a very small amount of food. Every calorie counts. Drinking unnecessary calories adds up even faster. Failure to avoid unnecessary calories almost always results in the failure to lose weight.

Most successful calorie counters learn that not writing down calorie counts doesn't work. This failure invariably results in repetitive small errors in calorie consumption which, in turn, cause weight gain. Counting calories is a lifelong process for those who have always struggled for weight control.

Failure should not be an excuse to quit trying. Increasing efforts, without exception, will eventually lead to weight loss. No one can maintain weight with falling calorie counts. There is never a guarantee that hard work will result in financial gain. But hard work dieting eventually results in weight loss.

People have different ideas as to what weight loss goals should be. Just about any weight loss can prove helpful. However, maintaining weight loss is even more important that achieving weight loss goals.

Lifelong dieting makes weight control last a lifetime!

Most people gain weight with age. Achieving weights that existed prior to age 20 is usually not realistic. Increased fluid retention and sagging associated with aging can prevent people from achieving weights that were normal many years past.

It's easy to feel 18 when you are 18. If you want to feel 18 when you are 40, you have to work at it. Diet and exercise are hard work for most. Few find pleasure in this. Most will find pleasure in achieving the goal of improved health.

"Ideal" weight goals are easy to determine. You are at your correct weight when the thickness of your skin below the belly button is the same as on your forearm. This is called the pinch test. Some bellies are large without being fat. A belly can stretch with age. This sag may or may not respond to exercise (stomach crunches). Therefore, the correct goal is not girth **of** the belly but rather thickness of the skin **on** the belly. People refer to this as "love handles." Most people are not in love with those handles. The size of the buttocks is not very important.

Step 3

Staying young is a losing battle. Losing weight doesn't have to be. The means of changing are harder than the goal of change. New calorie counts have to be ruthlessly maintained. If good health is to be achieved in America, it will never be achieved in a hospital bed. We are what we eat... and most of us need to eat better.

FLUFFY IN GERMANY

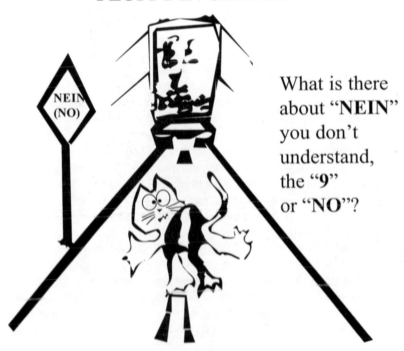

What is there about "**NEIN**" you don't understand, the "**9**" or "**NO**"?

Step 3

22. Carefully Counting with a Calorie Counter

Do you eat to live or do you live to eat? There is a difference. More than half of all Americans are overweight.

Determining what and how much food one should eat can be confusing. Nevertheless, losing weight can be self-taught with patience and perseverance. If you are overweight, you will need to change your diet. The correct way is very simple but hard work. The best way to avoid calories is to know where they are coming from. Accurate calorie counting is the foundation to weight control. Don't put food into your mouth unless you know how many calories it contains.

A calorie counter is set up like a dictionary. Instead of looking up a word to see what it means, you look up a food or drink to see how many calories it contains. Except water, everything has calories. A good calorie counter is as big as a desk dictionary. It's a book, not a pamphlet. All book stores sell these. All food labels contain this information as well.

Calories are listed by serving size (i.e. calories per ounces of food). Food and/or drink must be measured by weight or volume. Calories actually consumed are calculated by multiplying the calories per serving size by the portion consumed. Accurate calorie counts demand that all portions are weighed (food scales) or measured (measuring cups).

For example, if there are 100 calories in a 4-ounce serving, and you eat or drink 6 ounces, you will have taken in 150 calories. One hundred calories per 4 ounces multiplied by 6 ounces equals 150 calories ($100/4 \times 6 = 150$). In other words, (calories per serving size) X (serving size) = calories. Be sure the units of measurement of serving size are the same before and after the "X" (multiplication) sign. Many young people can help you with this math if you don't understand.

Homemade food dishes (e.g., casseroles) made with a variety of ingredients requires more complex math. Calories of all these separate foods need to be totaled in the dish prior to cooking. Once cooked, the dish needs to be weighed. Precooked total calorie count divided by the new cooked

Step 3

weight gives the calories per serving figure needed per portion. Don't guess your portion of this dish, weigh it!

Making and saving index cards of recipes with calorie counts per serving can prevent the need for duplicating these calculations. Many restaurants, especially chains (e.g., fast food), do these calculations for you on their menu items. When eating out, you can still count calories.

The human mind requires that all this information be written down or it will be forgotten. Write this information down before you eat it. Each day's calorie count should be totaled. At the end of each month, an average daily calorie count can be determined.

All of this hassle and work makes it easy to hate counting calories. Try to develop the same attitude about paperwork that you have about going to the bathroom. The job's not done until the paperwork's done! You might not *like* the paperwork but it's absolutely necessary. So why make a fuss?

Now look at your weight. Weigh yourself at the same time every day. Use an average for the week. Compare average weights with average calorie counts. If you are overweight and losing one to two pounds per week, you are eating the correct amount of calories. If not, you need to go up or down in your calorie intake. Do not lose more than two pounds a week; you will be losing muscle mass, not fat.

Once your correct calorie count is found, to maintain weight loss, you must eat this same number of calories every day for the rest of your life. This assumes your activity level stays the same. Failure to do so will allow the weight to return.

Dieting is never temporary. If there was no need to change your diet, why bother? If there was a need, why stop? "Eat to live" needs to last a lifetime.

Once you have determined what your calorie count should be, you must do everything in reverse. Calorie counting now determines portion size. You are looking up calories to see how much food you can eat (based on calories). This helps prevent overeating.

The biggest problem with a weight-losing diet is that the person may

Step 3

still feel hungry after eating the correct number of calories. Controlling hunger is a key ingredient to controlling total calorie intake. The solution is to find foods that are low in calories and high in fiber. High-fiber low-calorie foods can satisfy hunger (they are filling) and will not let you gain weight easily

Therefore, I recommend a calorie counter that also includes the fiber content of foods; most do not. Many foods that Americans eat don't have fiber and can't. Not everything you eat has to have fiber. But the goal is to eat the right food when fiber is an option. For example, you can eat an apple or drink apple juice. One has fiber and one doesn't. Here you have a choice. Always **eat** fruit; don't drink it.

Which do you think is better: Fruit Loops or Wheaties? The answer is neither! They are both "crap" and should be avoided. You cannot know whether any food is good without reading the label for calorie and fiber content.

There are many cereals you can choose from. You can find some that taste good and are good for you. In a calorie counter that also lists fiber (e.g., pictured at end of chapter), one can look up "Cereal; Ready-to-eat" and find approximately 350 cereals to pick from. Surely there are at least 10 low calorie, high fiber cereals you will like! (P.S. High-fiber bread and cereal are some of the best and easiest sources of fiber you can find.)

Most people on diets get into a rut of eating the same thing over and over again. This must be avoided so that you don't get tired of dieting. Successful dieting requires you to stop looking at old foods you cannot eat and find new foods you can eat. Once again, a calorie counter can help. In fact, you can start from the beginning of the book and go to the end, looking for low-calorie, high-fiber food items. Run your finger down two columns — calories and fiber. Stop and check out every item that meets these criteria. If it's something you like, eat it. If you don't know what it is, try it.

This strategy gives you many ideas of healthy things you can eat. By the time you get to the end of the calorie counter, you will have forgotten the beginning and you can start all over again. Variety is the spice of life. No one can eat the same thing every day. It will surprise you — how many things you can find to eat.

Many unadulterated high-fiber, low-calorie items taste bland. Some people think that cucumbers have this problem. Foods such as these can be seasoned. The pictured calorie counter lists over 400 salad dressings. Many of these are high in calories and should be avoided. But there are still over 50 to choose from. A cucumber can taste 50 different ways and we have not even gotten to carrots. Remember, dill pickles are also made from cucumbers (only 4 calories).

There are many low-calorie food flavorings and spices that can improve the taste of anything; you just need to learn how to use them. Many are pre-mixed and easy to use.

Dining out can be a caloric disaster. The last chapter of the pictured book lists many popular restaurants and fast food chains (look up your favorite one). You will be hard-pressed to find anything that is low in calories and high in fiber. Some appetizers served in restaurants exceed the caloric needs of an entire week's worth of food.

Simply put, if you want to lose weight, don't eat out. Pack your own lunch and make your own meals. It's safer to invite folks over for dinner than vice versa. If you do eat out, be very careful.

It's much easier to obtain information about calories and fiber from packaged foods by using their labels. This discourages calorie-counting dieters from using unpackaged food. That's a mistake. The more packaged a food is, the more likely someone added calories. Eat as close to the garden as possible.

Many packages make claims that their contents are better for you. "Lite" has become a popular word. The way to verify these claims is to compare that food item with others. This is cumbersome when shopping but can be done quickly using a calorie counter. All similar packages are grouped under one heading. By running your fingers down two columns (calorie count and fiber content), you can quickly ascertain what range of fiber and calories is possible in this category.

STEP 3

Obviously, in any category, you can pick and try the best products first (lowest calories and/or highest fiber). However, if you don't like the taste, you're not going to eat it for the rest of your life. So forget about it. Instead, try the second best one... and so on. Price, convenience, and availability also need to be considered.

But remember, a lot of calories is still a lot of calories. The lower range of calories (i.e. lite) in a high-calorie food item may still be too high. "Lite" ice cream is still fattening (and has no fiber) if it has lots of calories. You can't make chicken salad out of chicken crap.

You can't make real ice cream good for you if you are trying to lose weight. Cream is fat from milk. Remember, fat is always high in calories. (That's why dieters are interested in low-fat items, but don't bother counting fat grams. Counting calories will keep you away from high fat items.)

A calorie counter with a fiber content can be used in a variety of ways to help find foods that are both good and bad. All of this is meaningless if the food is not measured and the calorie count is not accurately done. There is no easy way to change and lose weight. It's a hard goal to achieve.

Obesity kills and many people die trying to lose weight. Diet pills, fad diet plans (always well-publicized), cocaine, and self-induced diseases will enable many to lose weight. These strategies are not safe long-term and, therefore, cannot be used as livelong remedies to obesity. You can't make chicken salad out of chicken crap.

There is no substitute for the right diet. If you want to safely lose weight, you must eat balanced meals with the right number of calories. The more fiber, the better. It's that simple.

P.S. Nutritional tips — Many people need to eat less red meat and more fish. Fish adds variety to a balanced diet. Please note that fish is not low in calories. Neither is skim milk. Water is what is needed to quench thirst. Milk is part of a meal. Calcium supplements have no calories for those who need extra calcium.

STEP 3

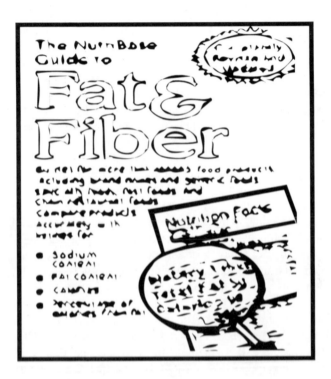

Calorie counting books, such as this one, are an excellent source of information about foods, their calories counts and fiber content. I am not endorsing this particular book (nor does this book endorse me) over others that offer the same information. This information is also available on CDs and the Web.

23. The Laws of Physics Apply to You Too

Did you know that physicians named themselves after "physicists"? Every branch of science contributes to our knowledge. Physicists helped build the most powerful electron microscopes in the world. No one brought us closer to our world than physicists. Physicists like precision. Physicists taught us the laws of physics. Physicists also invented quantum mechanics and the theory of relativity. Physicists examine particles so small that no one is even sure they exist. Physicists like to explain everything mathematically. Math is precise. The answer is either right or wrong... well, it used to be.

No one really understands physicists anymore...

A large amount of medical technology comes from physicists. They help invent and build x-ray machines, MRI scanners, lasers and computers. Where would medicine be without physicists? We have high expectations from modern medicine. Why not? If physicists can blow up the whole world with an atomic bomb, why can't physicians fix everything with the MRIs and computers that physicists have so kindly provided? Well, physicians can't. In medicine, the first step to staying alive is to stop killing yourself. Physicians are not physicists. We cannot change the laws of physics. Only physicists can!

But even physicists concede that precision has a price. Heisenberg was a physicist. Heisenberg's "uncertainty principle" ($[\text{delta}X][\text{delta}P] = [1.10^{-34} \text{ joules/second} \times (1/2)]$) is a mathematically precise answer to imprecision.

Huh?... It goes like this: as we study very small fast-moving particles, we cannot measure both position and speed. (That kinda' makes sense?) The more I concentrate on trying to find the little things, the less I notice how fast they are going. If I watch to see how fast these tiny particles are going, I won't see where they are. It's really a wonderful concept, precisely defining how wrong you can be. My dad is a physicist... So I became a physician. But like father, like son, I sometimes try to think like a physicist.

Living things are made up of many small food particles. We are what we eat when we can't eliminate those particles. When patients come to see

Step 3

me to stay well or to get well, I tell them to eat well. So-o-o what particular food particles do I recommend? That is a particularly difficult question to answer. (Dr. Heisenberg, stand aside.) This is why you need to understand "Dr. Meijer's uncertainty principle;" ("†s $f\mu\flat$—ˆç´®—=r.5)... Huh?... It goes like this: the more particular recommendations are about particular food particles, the more probable that they are wrong. (That kinda' makes sense?) Dietary advice can either be vaguely right or precisely wrong. It cannot be both.

Every nutritional label has precise percentages of daily vitamins and minerals recommended for a 2,000 calorie diet. Provided with such precise recommendations, you can be sure of one thing: they are wrong!

We are all made up of different food particles. Everyone doesn't need the exact same particular vitamins and minerals. Soooo..., even if it sounds precise, it doesn't mean that it is. The more precise the particulars are, the more the uncertainty is that those numbers are correct (which means they are wrong!).

On the other hand, some small dietary errors can cause big problems. Some people look at cake and gain weight. Since we are what we eat, it makes sense to take a look at the mirror. Our own measurements should help determine what and how many food particles we need.

Quantum medicine: both quality and quantity of little food particles are important.

Quality is hard to define. But the epidemic of cancer, kidney stones, gall bladder stones, heart attack, strokes, constipation, and diabetes gives us every indication that we are not eating the right kinds of food particles (quality). Quantity is much easier to figure out. Go weigh yourself. The epidemic of obesity indicates that the quantity of food particles can also be a problem. Because quantity can be precisely weighed, accurately counting calories can give predictable results. This is fortunate, since small errors in calories can cause big problems with weight.

"Dr. Meijer's certainty principle" (c=wt) is easier to understand: the longer you have been overweight, the more precisely you must count calo-

STEP 3

ries. Using calorie counts, we can eventually find the right quantity of food particles needed. But quality is much harder to define. All evidence points to some general recommendations. They are: the more fiber the better; using the USDA food pyramid as a guide for a balanced diet is reasonable; the closer to the garden you eat, the better; less meat, more fish. You can't make chicken salad out of .... Precise recommendations about vitamin E or polyunsaturated fats are as valuable as rockets to Mars... unless, of course, like a physicist, you want to go to Mars.

Dietary goals can be greatly influenced by a patient's goal. Goals for diabetics differ from Sumo wrestlers. Diabetics must eat 6 *teeny-weeny* meals per day; Sumo wrestlers must eat 6 **BIG-WIG** meals per day. Your physician can help you narrow your goals, but the more precise your particular goals are, the less likely you can correctly find the exact particular food particles you need ("Dr. Meijer's uncertainty principle"). Let's try this problem another way: if you were terminally ill, it would be natural for you to ask your doctor how long you might live. I can give you two answers: one is precisely wrong and the other, vaguely right. If I tell you that you will live 62 days, 32 minutes and 0.003 seconds, the answer is precise and most certainly wrong. Even if I shot you, you would not die at such a precise moment. If I tell you that you have 0 to 100 years, the answer is right but too vague to be helpful. It's not possible to precisely draw a line between these two unsatisfactory answers.

In quantum medicine, the price for precision on quality food particulars is uncertainty. Accept the limits of physicians, we are not physicists. Most patients aren't physicists, either. If you are overweight, weigh yourself. The laws of physics apply to you, too. Count calories because calories count.

24. The More They Know, the Less They Know

When confronted with serious illness, patients usually want only the best. For many people, the best doctors are the ones most specialized. "After all, that's all they do."

The best of the best are the ones who research and teach other doctors these specialized areas. The authors of new research are usually the names that surface when searching on the Web.

Common locations for famous researchers in medicine are the medical schools throughout the country. These doctors view themselves as the "experts" of their specialized fields. So do many other people.

Since all doctors were, at one time, medical students at one of these medical schools, all doctors have had contact with these experts. Like medical students, it's not uncommon for a doctor to look at these experts for guidance and advice. So here at these medical schools, sits and grows the great body of knowledge of medicine.

Experts form expert organizations, expert committees, expert societies, expert publications, expert research clinics, etc., etc. Experts quote other experts as references. No expert has to stand alone. There is a great body of expertise behind them.

These experts, like patients, want nothing but the best. Because their advice is so good, it should be heard. Many experts spend a considerable amount of time seeing to it that other doctors learn about their expert advice. In fact, experts actively publicize their advice by almost any means possible. They call their kind of advice "guidelines."

So, how are the experts doing?

To the dismay of experts, not all doctors and/or patients are heeding their expert advice (guidelines). In order to correct this problem, more and more experts find ways to actually impose their beliefs on others. "Guidelines" can be converted into government regulations. Insurance companies can be persuaded to only reimburse physicians who comply with expert guidelines. Finally, there is always the threat that an expert can testify against anyone who defies their expertise.

Many people forget that "the experts" went to the same medical schools as any other doctor. How a doctor becomes a researcher, teacher, etc., at a medical school varies. But suffice to say not all of the best doctors become researchers, teachers, etc. Many doctors who have never returned to medical school develop their own expertise in medicine without much fanfare.

Nevertheless, once an expert establishes his domain over fellow doctors, you can expect them to remain there. You can also expect more advice to be forthcoming.

One of the more dependable sources of "advice" is from the American Heart Association (AHA). They view themselves as the experts on heart disease. Because of this, they have established for us, very precisely, the correct way in which to try to revive a patient dying from a heart attack. These guidelines are called "Advance Cardiac Life Support" (ACLS) (i.e. the AHA way is the right way and any other way is the wrong way).

Naturally, the AHA has persuaded many hospitals, government regulators, etc., that physicians should revive patients in accordance with ACLS "guidelines."

To further ensure that physicians follow ACLS guidelines, more and more physicians are required to be certified by AHA as ACLS-trained. This means that physicians must memorize the "guidelines" that AHA experts have established.

Survival rates for patients whose hearts have stopped working due to heart attacks are low. Whatever improvement has been made is due to a machine commonly known as a defibrillator (it "shocks" the heart). CPR (cardiopulmonary resuscitation) is usually only helpful if a defibrillator can be used within 10-15 minutes.

There has never been any evidence that the rest of the ACLS guidelines have done anything to improve survival rates. In fact, techniques similar to today's CPR existed many years ago. These old techniques failed to save patient lives because back then there were no defibrillators to follow up on

Step 3

these techniques. Because no patient survived, these techniques were presumed to be ineffective and were abandoned.

Today's CPR is carefully defined by the "guidelines" of the AHA. Now there is "a right way" to do CPR and everything else is the wrong way. Nevertheless, it's likely that past techniques were probably as effective as the scientific babble that the AHA issues today as CPR "guidelines." Again, being CPR certified is becoming more and more a requirement for physicians. (Trivial questions about CPR were included on my board exam.)

In the meantime, ACLS standards are continuously being updated. Some current recommendations totally contradict previous ones. Other old recommendations quietly disappear. A lot of the new standards of ACLS do not resemble the old ones. Nevertheless, the new standards have to be memorized just like the old ones need to be forgotten in order to remain ACLS-certified.

All these certificates are demanded even though there is still no solid evidence that ACLS has ever increased the survival rates of patients. Many people use defibrillators without ACLS guidelines. Their results are just as good as those from physicians who are badgered into submitting to ACLS "guidelines."

The older I get, the more I see that the "experts" in medicine are not so right after all. The more specific and dogmatic they are with their "guidelines," the more likely they will have to retract that advice. Some experts are so specialized in their field of medicine that they obviously cannot see past their own noses. In any event, I am really starting to realize how cumbersome and irrelevant expert advice can be.

If anyone can make a mountain out of a molehill, it's an expert on a committee issuing guidelines. Experts are not the best or the worst in the medical profession. They are just doctors like the rest of us. They certainly aren't any better than the rest of us.

At the risk of tooting my own horn, I think it's time people appreciate the expertise of many less-recognized physicians. Your own doctor can sometimes be your best "expert" on what you need to do. The prominent

STEP 3

influence that organized legal experts (e.g., AHA) have, does not mean their advice is better than your own doctor's.

Sometimes common sense will have to be the better judge.

Difficult illnesses can be frustrating but if I get sick, I don't plan to run to the Web. More times than not, new ideas do not stand the test of time. Any new treatment is not always better than older treatments (or even no treatment). I personally feel that the best advice is usually the advice that has been around the longest. I plan to settle for a lot of good, old-fashioned advice from doctors I know personally.

A lot of "guidelines" aren't worth the paper they are printed on. One idea rarely works for the whole world. The more experts think they know what the whole country should do, the less they know.

Do I have a beef with experts? YEAH!

They keep giving my patients and me bad advice... and more and more people are subjected to "guidelines" that have been converted into regulations or hospital policy. One way or the other, experts want us to obey...cuz' they said so.

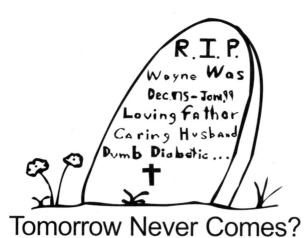

Tomorrow Never Comes?

25. Golly, Different Types of Diabetics Have Different Types of Problems

There are two types of diabetes, Type 1 and Type 2.

Type 1 diabetics commonly develop their disease before adulthood. Since this disease does not run in families, it strikes from nowhere. The need for insulin is immediate. Children with diabetes Type 1 can be very sick (so much for childhood).

Type 1 represents less than 5% of all diabetics. When these young diabetics become teenagers, they usually rebel against authority, resulting in poor sugar control. Young diabetics yearn to live a normal life like their peers. But by young adulthood, many are already suffering from complications caused by their disease.

Type 2 diabetes is much more common. These patients have lived a normal life until they developed their diabetes. In fact, it's normal in America to be overweight with poor dietary habits, which are the most common reasons these diabetics develop Type 2. By the time diabetes develops, many other problems associated with obesity and diabetes may have already developed. Type 2 diabetics simply add this problem to their lists of common ailments.

Both types of diabetics face dietary issues. But the concerns differ considerably. Type 2 diabetics tend to be overweight and have been on and off diets for years. These patients tend to skip the six recommended meals and are always trying to "cut back." Type 1 diabetics are not usually overweight, but they have had severe episodes of hypoglycemia (low sugar). To prevent passing out from hypoglycemia and wrecking their cars, Type 1 diabetes avoid under-eating or skipping any meals.

The older diabetics are, the more their medical problems grow. But the list for Type 2 diabetics usually differs from Type 1.

The early list of problems for Type 1 diabetics is almost always related to their disease. This includes blindness, kidney failure, infertility (or impotence), and polyneuropathy (the common cause of amputations).

STEP 3

Early on, but at a later age, Type 2 diabetics struggle with high cholesterol, arthritis, obesity, hypertension, and even perhaps a heart attack.

Type 1 diabetics tend to see endocrinologists (doctors who specialize in diabetes) as their primary care doctor. All their medical problems are related to diabetes. Type 2 diabetics tend, on the other hand, to see internists or family practitioners for a wide range of problems.

Diet causes, prevents, and treats Type 2 diabetes. The importance of diet is irrefutable and the changes needed, undeniable. Oral medication (pills) can also be added to treatment. Type 1 diabetics, especially with insulin pumps, may or may not require dietary improvements. Diet does not cause the disease. Complex insulin regimes trying to maintain fragile blood sugar control are the cornerstone of treatment for Type 1 diabetics.

It's easy to see why these two different types of diabetes can create very different issues. But other differences can develop between diabetic patients. Factors such as education or wealth can also influence problems for diabetics.

Rich diabetics struggle more trying to diet (they can eat out too much and many restaurants are caloric disasters) than buying medication. Poor patients worry more about buying medication than trying to diet. Patients who can read have an easier time trying to control their diabetes than those who can't.

One of the most popular concepts in medical care is to improve quality of care by establishing "standards of care." No one loves to establish "standards of care" for diabetics more than the American Diabetic Association (ADA).

However, not all diabetics are the same. Type 1 and Type 2 are clearly two different diseases. It's never made sense to me why these two diseases are subjected to the same ADA "standards of care" or served by the same organization. (It's like the Lung Association taking care of heart patients.)

People and diseases are different. Doctors are different, too. Has anyone really proven that differences in care are such a bad thing? I doubt it. Individualized medical care really makes more sense. One size does *not* fit all.

STEP 3

Educated patients (patients who understand their disease) can really help their doctors tailor their goals to their individual needs. Educated patients do not need a degree in medicine. Patient education is what you know about your disease. Goals are what you want. Education improves the goals and the means.

That's what this book is all about — educating patients. Better educated patients have proven to get better results. That's because they are getting both what they need and what they want. Once educated, both patients and doctors need to create priority lists. You cannot do everything at the same time.

Doctors' priority lists and patients' priority lists are never the same. Just as the perspective for Type 1 and Type 2 diabetes is so different, so is the perspective between doctors and patients. Being different isn't wrong; it's just more complicated. The complexity of good medical care rarely makes "standards of care" wholly applicable to many patients (when has a square peg fit into a round hole?).

Unfortunately, educated patients usually discover that they are part of the problem. It's always a rude discovery to realize that no one is perfect, including you. Doctors make mistakes, too. This means there can never be perfect medical care... just good care. So don't look back too long at mistakes. Instead, become part of the solution. The best medical care always includes an educated patient. Once educated, patients can usually set better goals than those set by others.

If you need to learn something new, let your doctor know.

Step 3

26. Y'all Void' Missing a Meal Now, Yuh Hear?

In plain English, here are some tips to avoid hypoglycemia. Remember?, ...when you run out of gas, you run out of go... don't remember? Reread the second chapter of this book... **N-O-W!!!**

TIPS:

1. Keep canned fruit/food (low calorie, high fiber) in the car, office, etc. for unexpected emergencies. Some require can openers, some do not. If it is a severe emergency, drink the juice and eat the fruit. Otherwise, drain the juice. Some stores sell canned fruit without any added sweeteners. Look for these (read the label).

2. Dried fruit (raisins, apricots) is small, high in fiber, and high in calories. Unlike candy, nutritious. In a baggy, small and very portable.

3. A small electronic food timer/alarm can easily be set for the next meal time. People with poor vision or arthritis can use these. Many can attach on clothing.

4. On trips, always plan for two unexpected delays that prevent you from arriving to your next two meals.

5. Any food store has fast food that is more nutritious than any fast-food restaurant.

6. Unusually long or active days require extra calories. More small snacks of fruit (e.g., raisins), food, etc. work better than bigger meals. Drink water, period.

7. Some candy bars have fiber. Some breakfast bars are worse than candy. Rare emergencies will require candy bars for fuel... any food is better than no fuel.

8. If something delayed your meal and nothing happened, figure it can happen again and you might not be so lucky next time. An honest mistake happens once, not twice. A fatal mistake is the last one. Plan to fix all your mistakes, ...*after* the first time they occur.

9. Diabetics who work outside a lot for long periods of time need big

STEP 3

pockets. Vehicles can carry 12V DC power converters (to 120V AC) to power microwaves (<800 watts) at construction sites. Hot fast meals to go?

10. There never is a good reason to skip a meal, just poor planning or a dumb mistake, but nobody is perfect. Practice makes perfect.

11. Food is food. Breakfast food can be eaten for dinner and vice-versa. Cereal can be eaten without milk Anything hot can be cold.

12. Almost any leftover will keep for 2 hours in your pocket, one advantage of a small meal.

13. You can't give an excuse that someone else hasn't already given and fixed. Solutions are there, you just haven't learned them yet. Quit telling us what you can't do, find what you can do. Trying doesn't count. Good excuses don't fix problems.

14. God made microwaves for diabetics who need fast food while on the road, at work, or in a hurry. Small microwaves fit in travel bags and at the office. Power converters in cars, boats, or campers can produce enough power for a small microwave. Buy a small refrigerator. You figure out the rest...

15. One big meal can be divided into 2 small meals, one bigger meal can be divided into 3 small meals, one feast can be divided into 4 small meals, one bigger feast can be divided into 5 small meals, one banquet can be divided into 6 small meals, etc.... won't you sing your A, B, C's with me?... using a calorie counter for new ideas to eat?...

16. Frozen peas can serve as a small ice-bag for a bottle of water. Half-frozen peas can also be microwaved and served....got peas and water to go, so ah' void' missin' uh' meal now. Shuck's, how bout' some corn instead?

> # If you have a brain, why not use it before you put something in your mouth?

Step 3

27. *STEP 3* for Control of Diabetes

You cannot have your cake and eat it too. Here are your choices — you only live to eat or you only eat to live. You can't do both. Today is the third step towards *your control* of diabetes.

Goals for STEP 3:

A. Learn how many calories you're eating. You must buy food scales, read and follow the directions of *22. Carefully Counting with a Calorie Counter.* Try to reread these directions at least once a day. You might be working on Step 3 for more than one office visit. A lot of mistakes and problems can occur here. Your doctor will not judge you by how many mistakes you make. We all make mistakes. Instead, he will assess the effort you make. Your doctor's ability to help you is determined by your effort to help yourself. No one can do this for you. Practice makes perfect. Start today, not tomorrow. Read *21. The Means and the Goal* the night before your next office visit.

B. Eat less but more often. Remember a diabetic needs six meals per day. Eat a little of a lot rather than a lot of a little.

C. Exercise is important. You need to be thinking about an exercise program. Read *36. Dying to Run.*

Questions commonly asked by patients:

How many calories should I eat? We still don't know exactly how many calories you should eat. This will be determined in future steps (don't get ahead of us). For now, from what you have already learned, use common sense to decide how much you should eat, eat it, and count the calories of these meals. There is no "right" answer. Make sure you write down whatever you are doing.

Do I always have to count calories (every time!)? Yes. For long-

Step 3

term   control of diabetes, it is essential that you determine what your calorie count is now and later. Over time, if you live long enough, your diabetes will get worse (i.e. harder to control blood glucose). To maintain control over your diabetes, your diet will have to get better over time. We have that time.   It was not your decision to become a diabetic. It is beyond your control that your diabetes will get worse (harder to control sugar) over time. What you can do is maintain normal blood glucose (sugar) levels. This can be done with improved diet and medication over time. Time does not stand still. Neither should you. You will spend the rest of your life improving the way you eat (and later exercise).

How can I count calories eating out? Menus and restaurants can sometimes provide caloric information. See also the back section of your calorie counter (book). There is no law against measuring food with food scales and/or measuring cups in a restaurant or at a friend's house. It is legal and moral. Calorie counting must be done (or don't eat out).

Why are there diabetics who don't count calories? Remember whose funeral you want to attend — yours or theirs? Life is not fair but there are still many things worth living for. Grow old dieting or die a lot younger — the choice is yours. Remember, the longer you have struggled with obesity or diabetes (in other words, the more you hate dieting), the more precisely you have to count calories and eliminate crap.

Can I eat any sugar or fat? If you know something is high in sugar or fat, you shouldn't eat it. This is especially true for plain table sugar (sucrose) and added caloric sweetener. Not all "sugar" is sucrose. Blood glucose is "sugar." Many healthy foods naturally contain some kind of sugar and/or fat. The total elimination of dietary fat or sugar is not possible since most foods contain some amounts of these things. The goal is to reduce, not eliminate, sugar and fat (especially plain table sugar-sucrose). How? Eat less calories. Eat things that have fiber in it. Don't drink calories (except milk for cereal).

Can I use sugar substitutes as much as I want? Artificial sweeteners (sugar substitutes) are not nutritious. Maintaining and satisfying a "sweet

Step 3

tooth" is an invitation for more temptation. A diabetic needs to eat what is good for health, not what simply tastes good. If it tastes good and it is good for you (fruit) GREAT! If it tastes good but is not nutritious (i.e. good for you) — FORGET IT. No crap. Calorie-wise, a diet soda is better than a "regular" soda. But God only knows what other crap is in a diet soda. If you are thirsty, all you need is water. Water has no calories and it is the only thing really needed when you are thirsty. Again, **no** crap.

THERE IS NO EVIDENCE THAT ARTIFICIAL SWEETENERS ARE HELPING AMERICANS TO LOSE WEIGHT. It is strongly recommended you avoid all artificial sweeteners (e.g., diet sodas).

Questions for you!!!!

Do you know what the leading cause of non-traumatic amputation is?
Diabetes.
Do you know what the leading cause of preventable blindness is?
Diabetes.
Do you know what the leading cause of kidney failure (dialysis) is?
Diabetes.
Do you know what the leading cause of death is in diabetics?
Heart attack.
Do you know how to prevent amputations, blindness, dialysis, impotence, heart attacks, strokes, etc, etc.... in a diabetic?
Diet, diet, diet, diet, diet, diet...
Do you know how to double insulin sensitivity in Type 2 diabetics?
Lose 5 lbs.
What does the body really need (crave for) when thirsty?
Water (not soda).

Questions your doctor might ask you:

Do you know all your medication bottles?

STEP 3

Do you want to end up having an amputation?
(In other words, are you counting calories?)
What are you having trouble with (diet, weight, or sugar)?
What did you eat on _____ ? (any day of the week)
What time did you eat that?
How many calories was that?
Did you have any hypoglycemic (low sugar) reactions?
Why did you skip meals?
What do you believe is your average calorie count per day?
Do you have any questions or concerns?

EAT   FRUIT
DON'T DRINK IT

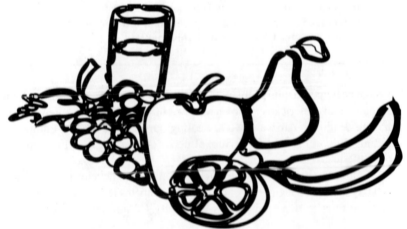

STEP 4

28. If Losing Weight Was So Easy, There Wouldn't Be So Many Fat People

> **THE QUIZ**
> What does watching football have in common with watching baseball?
> What does a bar mitzvah have in common with a baptism?
> What does a funeral have in common with a wedding?
> What does Christmas have in common with Thanksgiving?
> What does a billboard have in common with television?
> What does breakfast have in common with dinner?
> What does a birthday have in common with New Year's Day?
> What do planes have in common with trains?
> What does Mother's Day have in common with Easter?
> What does Valentine's Day have in common with Halloween?
> What does going to the movies have in common with going to a circus?
> What does a wedding anniversary have in common with a family reunion?
> What does a country fair have in common with a city festival?
> What does the Fourth of July have in common with Labor Day?
> Answers for QUIZ at end of this chapter.

The biggest health problem looming in America today is obesity. More than half of all Americans are overweight. In poor countries, many people starve to death. In America, we are eating ourselves to death. Eating and drinking without regard for nutritional needs is catching up with more and more Americans.

Obesity can increase the chance for someone to develop diabetes more than sixty fold. The incidence of obesity and diabetes has increased so much that some refer to this epidemic as "diabesity." The more you eat like an

Step 4

American, the more likely you will die like one.

Many people seeking medical care want to stay young and healthy. Most patients do not want to die. It's pretty amazing that the majority of diseases we see are at least partially self-inflected. It's not that death isn't inevitable. It's just that we tend to speed it up. Rarely do any of us die without lending a hand to our own demise.

"To err is human..." Part of the problem with diseases is our difficulty in correcting problems that we are responsible for creating. It never would have been a problem if it were easy to change. Smokers with bad lungs find it hard to stop smoking; alcoholics find it hard to stop drinking; and overweight people find it hard to lose weight.

Mistakes are unavoidable. We are all guilty of doing stupid things. There is no cure for stupidity. Doing dumb things doesn't mean you are stupid. Everyone makes dumb mistakes. The fact that the majority of Americans eat improperly is another example of how stupid we all can be (myself included).

When the overwhelming majority of people make the same dumb mistakes, it becomes difficult to recognize that what they are doing is stupid. America is the fattest country in the world and it's getting fatter faster. The need for physicians to counsel patients about their diet and lack of exercise will increase. More and more patients need to be told that what they are doing will harm themselves.

No one needs to be condemned for being human.

Condemn the mistake, not the person who made it. Without condemnation, there can be no motive for change. But to get better, patients have to be part of the solution.

Physicians diagnose and treat disease. When possible, we prescribe medications to patients to treat their illnesses. Pills that work provide proof to the old adage that "we are what we eat."

Medication is the most potent example of how food and drink can affect our health. It should come to no surprise to anyone that excessive amounts of the wrong food and drink will cause problems. Other bad "hab-

STEP 4

its" (e.g., cigarettes, alcohol, etc.) are also things that we put in our mouths.

It's very common that while the physician is trying to get the patient better, the patient isn't (trying). Too much fat, sugar and protein without enough fiber clearly contributes to all the important diseases in America. ("Common things occur commonly.")

Because patients can choose what goes into their mouths, teaching patients lifestyle changes (diet, stop smoking, etc.) are all important components of treating many diseases. I always tell patients that the first step to getting better (treatment) is to stop killing yourself. A pill cannot fix what you put in your own mouth.

Therefore, a good physician is also a good teacher. Good patients are good students, willing to learn and change destructive behavior. Since both are human, neither is expected to be perfect. But the effort needs to be there.

No one depends solely on the doctor to decide what goes into his/her mouth. The majority of what we eat and drink is taught by the society in which we live, not medicine.

In a democracy where the majority rules, it can be hard for a patient to remember what a physician has taught him or her. Nevertheless, it always matters why you eat, what you eat and how much you eat. The patient, not the doctor, pays the price for failure.

Historically, preventing self-inflicted disease has always been a difficult task. Nevertheless, America has been successful in increasing the number of smokers who have stopped smoking. This success can be expected. In the past, tobacco companies were successful in increasing the number of people who smoked. If we can change in the *wrong* direction, we can also change in the *right* direction.

We don't have solutions for all problems. Some problems, like dumb mistakes, never seem to go away. But there should be solutions for any problem that is changing and becoming worse. If we are doing things to make obesity more common and severe, we can also do things to make it better.

For modern medicine to be successful in providing Americans with

STEP 4

good health, not only do patients have to take medications as prescribed, they must learn from their doctor what they need to do to help make themselves better. A lot depends on what you put in your mouth. You can only feel as good as you eat.

The answer is the same for each "QUIZ" question: food and drink!

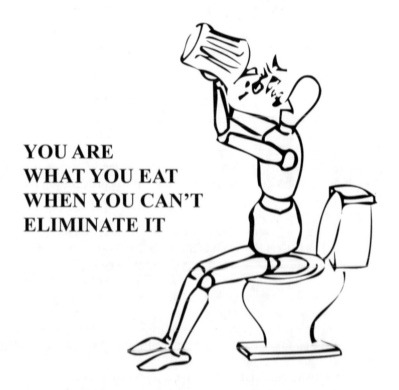

**YOU ARE
WHAT YOU EAT
WHEN YOU CAN'T
ELIMINATE IT**

Sweet tea is water with brown crap in it.

Step 4

29. Dumb Diet Questions/Answers for Dummies Like Me

Doc says, "More fiber, less calories." How do you know how many calories to eat? Weigh yourself. You are eating too many calories if you are too heavy and not losing weight or you are gaining weight. One exception to this rule: fluid from swelling can also change your weight.

What is my right weight? You're probably at the right weight when the thickness of your skin on your forearm is the same (as thin) as the skin around your belly button. (It's called the pinch test.) Big butts may be okay and do not cause much concern from a health point of view.

What's fiber? It's plant material that is not digested and comes out at the other end. Examples include the string in celery sticks, the wood in trees, the pulp of fruit, and seeds.

Why is fiber important? Diets high in fiber reduce your chances of heart attack, stroke, and cancer by one half. We don't know why. It could be something that is simply associated with fiber. In addition, fiber is filling and satisfies hunger. Since fiber is not digested, it has no calories and helps people (trying to lose weight) eat fewer calories. It prevents constipation and diarrhea. It helps diabetics control blood sugar. It has been proven to prevent diabetes. (Does that run in your family?) How much fiber should I eat? As far as we know, the more the better.

Are all plant foods good for you? No. Besides some plants that are poisonous, you can eat too much of plants that are high in calories. Starches are plants. But potatoes and corn are also high in calories. Some starches have little fiber (potato). The shell of a kernel of corn has fiber; you can see those come out at the other end. But the inside contents of a kernel of corn is high in calories and has no fiber.

How much fiber is there in meat (protein)? Meats, eggs and dairy products have no fiber. Fat has no fiber. Only beans have protein *and* fiber. Remember, beans are plant seeds.

Do you recommend a vegetarian diet? There is still heated debate on this but I personally do not recommend a vegetarian diet. An egg or a small piece of meat (the size of an egg) offers a wide variety of nutrients that are difficult to obtain on a pure vegetarian diet. Most Americans eat too much protein and not enough fish.

What's "sugar"? Normal people think of this as table sugar. This white granule is made from sugar cane (which is a plant). The "cane" that has fiber is separated from its starchy content that can be "purified" into table sugar. Sugar tastes sweet and its use is popular because of this. Other plants can be used to provide high concentrations of sweeteners. A common sweetener is corn syrup. From a medical point of view, all these "sugars" are the same: high in calories with no fiber content. Refined caloric sweeteners lack essential nutrients. All plants contain sugar. There is no such thing as a "sugar-free diet." The difference between table sugar and something like fruit is the degree to which the "sugar" has been separated from all fiber and become concentrated in calories without any nutrients. This "purification" removes valuable vitamins, minerals, etc. Sweet whole fruit is OK for diabetics to eat, but how many can't be ignored. Eat fruit, don't drink it.

Can you give me specific examples of good food to eat? Let's start with breakfast. Eggs? One egg is not high in calories, is inexpensive, and provides high quality protein, minerals and vitamins. Most people do not need more than one egg per day. Grits (South Carolinian question)? Sorry... not so good. It's simply corn without fiber (like sugar), @!!*# Cereal? I'll get to that.. Sausage biscuit (SC question)? The answer is a big fat **NO**! That has more fat and calories than a Big Mac. Biscuits have no fiber.

Coffee? Decaffinated is water with brown crap in it. Caffeine can cause heartburn, insomnia, irregular heartbeats and can be highly addictive. If you are thirsty, drink water.

Cereal? Read the label; find ones with high fiber and low calories. Many people are surprised to learn that Wheaties and corn flakes do not have fiber. Many high fiber cereals have more added sugar than Fruit Loops or Lucky Charms. Again, read the label. On the other hand, many high fiber, low calorie cereals taste like cardboard. One simple solution is to mix two high fiber cereals together. Add a little bit of a tasty high fiber, high calorie cereal to the low-calorie one (that tastes like cardboard). Another example of how to improve cereal is with raisin bran. It's high in fiber, but all brands have raisins covered with added sugar. The solution here is to buy high fiber flakes and mix it with your own dried (e.g., raisins) or fresh fruit. Simply put, make your own raisin bran.

Lunch? Avoid fast food. Fast food tends to be high protein, high fat (meat) with no fiber (including white bread), and soda (flavored water with sugar). All this is very high in calories and without fiber, the main problem with a typical American diet. What can I eat? There are frozen foods that are low in calories and can be microwaved. High fiber bread and crackers can be used to make sandwiches. Fruit and vegetables can be added. How about supper? Restaurants, like fast foods, serve high protein, high fat with very small portions of vegetables. High fiber bread is also hard to come by. If you must eat out, buy a main entree with extra plates. Divide this up with your party. Drink water. Take the money you save and buy a large number of side orders of vegetables, salads, and high fiber bread. The end result is not a cheaper meal (side orders are expensive)...just a healthier one (a patient taught me this idea). What's wrong with artificial sweeteners (Nutrasweet, diet sodas, etc., etc.)? At the very best, these things are harmless. No one has ever suggested that these have any nutritional value. The average American eats a pound of this stuff every five days. Could this not be harmful? I think there is evidence that artificial sweeteners could be harmful to the nervous system (that's brains). There is no evidence that these products reduce sugar consumption, an increasingly worse problem for America. Eating what is good for you beats dying young.

YOU CAN ONLY FEEL
AS GOOD
AS YOU EAT

Step 4

30. Dieters on the Run

Eating "on the run," every day, Americans stand in line waiting for "fast food." Many eat fast food trying to save time. Eating out, especially fast food, is a caloric and nutritional disaster. Despite all of our running around, we have become the fattest country in the world.

Dieting, especially for weight control, requires the time needed to prepare one's own foods. Eating out needs to be avoided but a lot of dieters complain that they don't have time to maintain their own diet. They, too, need to eat "on the run."

The answer to the problem about time is to make better use of time. College graduates call planning ahead "time management."

Planning ahead can find improvements based on past mistakes and future needs. Planning ahead helps to break old bad habits (e.g., standing in line for "fast food"). Planning ahead can eliminate wasted time (e.g., standing in line for "fast food").

The hardest part about dieting is not actually time. It's getting in the habit and remembering to plan ahead. The fact is that any meal requires planning. The difference between real planning and last minute planning is **when** you plan and whether there is enough time to do anything sensible.

To make matters worse, a lot of last-minute meal plans could have been done faster if the meal had been planned days ahead.

Either way, it's no surprise that we need to take time to eat. If not, we starve to death. It's not **if** you are going to make plans, it's when. One can even plan when to plan ahead. Some of my best planning occurs in traffic jams (commuting). Good ideas can be saved using common technology. You can call your own voice mail via cell phone and leave a message for tomorrow's grocery list. There are many variations to this basic idea. You can use a tape recorder at a stop light instead of a cell phone in a traffic jam.

Think before you eat. Better eating comes from better ideas. One better idea is planning ahead (improved time management).

One of my favorite time savers is the microwave. Microwaves have become very inexpensive. An extra one at work is very affordable. You can get a 12-volt adapter and operate one in your car. Any time, any place, you can quickly microwave a fast meal. So what can you make? Well, microwave cookbooks usually come with microwaves. The recipes in these books are short and easy. Frozen dinners have greatly improved in both quality and choices. Most have easy microwave directions. These little ideas can be added to a growing list of "fast food" you can make and eat.

You can deliberately make "leftovers." Be sure you don't eat these extra portions when you are already full. There are a lot of inexpensive, disposable ways to preserve food (e.g., freezer bags). A small fridge at work is not expensive. Later, you can use prepackaged utensils with napkins to accompany disposable plates, bowls, cups, etc., to make another fast meal.

Encourage fellow workers to picnic with you rather than invite you to eat out. Help form an exercise group for lunch breaks.

In other words, make plans to build your own fast food restaurant that is conveniently located in your own home, car, work, "on the run," etc. Most of the time, you will find that your fast food is cheaper than that served at restaurants. The art of making your own lunch has been greatly eroded by the attitude that "no one has time to make lunch at home." The time wasted standing in line for fast food usually goes unnoticed. Nothing is faster than eating your own lunch at work. Time lost at home is easily made up at work. So what is there to do with an hour-long lunch break? If need be, you can stand in line (eating) at the grocery store to buy next week's lunches rather than standing in line waiting to eat.

A lot of junk food is eaten as quick snacks. Planned snacks are better and can be just as quick. In order to eat fresh fruit, you have to plan on when to buy it and when to eat it. A boiled egg requires the prior thought of when to boil it. Any of these examples are much better than a bag of chips or a candy bar. Many planned items are also cheaper (e.g., an egg).

If shelf life or food storage is a problem, planning can help again. Canned fruit (no sugar or artificial sweeteners added) and dried fruit (e.g.,

Step 4

raisins, dried apricots, etc.,) are snacks with long shelf lives where spoilage is much less of an issue. Raisins can be carried in a shirt pocket or purse. Canned food can be stored anywhere near a can opener. (A quick unplanned snack they may be!)

A lot of time is spent cleaning up when we prepare our own meals. Planning can also shorten cleanup time. Recipes for one pot meals can save a lot of mess. Using a gas grill outside can reduce mess inside. Disposable aluminium pans, aluminum foil, ovenproof bags and plastic wrap reduce cleanup time. Finally, like a fast food restaurant, any and all utensils and plates can be disposable. All this disposable material may seem expensive, but they are not per meal. If McDonalds can afford it, why can't you? If your time is money, saving time also saves money. Fast food at home can be as fast as fast food away from home. It's just that home food, with planning, can be healthier (if you so choose).

Many new large food stores are being built that have extensive delis. These areas are usually loaded with quick new ideas for meals. Some stores will also allow you to eat there. It's high class fast food with better selections. It's also new ideas that you can use at home. (Just be sure to read the label before you buy or eat it.)

Many food stores understand that dieters don't have time to waste. Stores now sell fresh vegetables that are adequately washed and can be eaten right out of the package. Just plan on having the right utensils when you need them.

Food stores also offer a lot of ideas on improving food flavoring. A lot of seasonings are now packaged for speed and convenience. These improvements usually include microwave directions. Cooked chicken can taste a hundred different ways using a hundred different packages to season it. Also, look for packages that say, "Add chicken."

When you can't think of something to eat, go through your calorie counter from "A" to "Z." As you run your finger down two columns (calories and fiber), you can find many low calorie, high fiber foods you could consider eating.

STEP 4

The cost of packaging fast food can sometimes exceed the cost of the food. (Haste makes waste.) But you can save a lot of time. Furthermore, you can spend less money by not having to eat out. Don't forget to also consider the medical costs of a bad diet from traditional fast food.

Poor planning is usually the cause of failing to improve or maintain needed dietary changes. It doesn't have to be. Excuses about cost and time can be overcome if new ideas replace old bad habits. There is a great deal of technology out there that can save you time and money. Dieters on the run can keep up with anyone else. Remember, your feet cannot outrun your hands! Dietary goals, such as weight control, are totally dependent on eliminating the diet that caused your problems in the first place. Time is money, but money can't buy everything. Times change from time to time; fools don't.

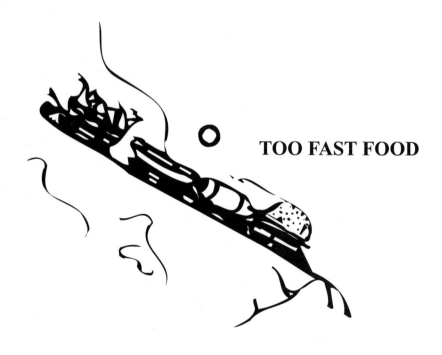

TOO FAST FOOD

STEP 4

31. LOOK WHO'S TALKING

Some organizations get so big the "right hand doesn't know what the left hand is doing." Companies with thousands of employes have this problem. Imagine the communication problems of a company with a half million employees.

The human body is a very complex organization made up of many, many cells. In order for us to stay alive, our cells must communicate with each other. How can you function if you don't know what either hand is doing?

A stroke is a communication problem between your brain and your hand. Paralysis can be caused by the brain's inability to generate the signals needed for communication. The nerve (wire) needed to carry the message could be cut as well. The failure of the arm to listen can also cause paralysis.

It's not practical for every single muscle cell to have its own nerve ending (wire). To reduce the number of wires sent from the brain to the muscle, one muscle cell can pass the message on to another to help move the arm. Failure of the muscle cells to communicate with each other can also cause paralysis. Finally, dead or broken muscle cells don't move (another cause of paralysis).

Identifying where the problem is (e.g., paralysis) obviously helps to narrow down what the problem could be. Many medical tests do just that. These tests determine where, not what, the problem is. Even if the ultimate cause cannot be determined, knowing where the problem is can suggest solutions. In some instances, that's enough to begin treatment.

A very efficient way for cells to communicate with each other over long distances is with hormones. A hormone is a chemical substance that is usually produced by a small cluster of cells (gland). When other cells, that are the intended recipients, come in contact with the hormone, a message is delivered by its presence.

Transmitting information like this is not new. Before telephones were invented, smoke signals were used to transmit messages over long distances.

Step 4

One only had to agree beforehand what the presence of smoke would mean. Many people, not just one person, could be the recipient of the message yet only one person had to build a fire.

Birth control pills are hormones that create a lot of smoke for the reproductive system. This smoke causes miscommunication between the cells that make up the reproductive system. The failure to maintain normal communication within the reproductive system prevents the coordination needed for the possibility of pregnancy. In this case, disruption of communication between cells is the goal.

Usually miscommunications cause problems, not solutions.

The thyroid gland produces a hormone called thyroid hormone (that's a clever name). Every cell in the body is like a little motor. These motors cannot be turned off. Dead motors mean dead cells. They can either run wide open or idle when not being used. Thyroid hormone controls the idle adjustment. If thyroid hormone is high (hyperthyroidism), the motor will idle faster than normal; if set too low, the cell will idle too slowly (and possibly turn off, resulting in death).

Some hormones are much more important than others. Some are "heard" by every cell in the body. It doesn't sound like much of a job for thyroid hormone to set the idle adjustment of every cell. But if every single cell in the body idles too fast, a lot of fuel is wasted.

"Low thyroid" is called hypothyroidism. If thyroid hormone is low, every cell will idle slower and slower until the motor finally turns off. In other words, failure to take prescribed thyroid replacement is a fatal mistake.

Most people think of estrogen when "hormones" are mentioned. Many do not recognize that insulin is also a hormone. However, insulin affects different cells in different ways. Some cells take blood glucose in while others release glucose (i.e. same messenger, different message). However, the cumulative effect of insulin is always the same — as insulin levels fall, blood glucose levels rise.

Every motor depends on the correct mixture of fuel and air, via the carburetor, to run properly. Too much fuel "floods" the motor. A motor

STEP 4

stops when it runs out of gas.

Insulin is the carburetor for every cell in the body. It's supposed to mix the right amount of fuel with the right amount of air. Too much blood glucose, every cell has a flooded motor. Low blood glucose (hypoglycemia), the cells start to run out of gas.

The ability of hormones to affect so many cells' behavior can either prove helpful or cause disease. These chemicals not only affect the behavior of many individual cells, but the cumulative effect of these affected cells has impact too (e.g., high blood glucose levels).

Without hormones, there would be a tremendous lack of coordination between cells. The need for this communication should be obvious. It is the combined and coordinated efforts of the heart, lung, red blood cells, and blood vessels that allow fuel and air to be delivered to every cell in the body. Blood not only carries many essential nutrients, it also carries many essential messages. Different cells listen to and respond to different hormones.

Medications can mimic hormones. If a drug can behave like a hormone, a small amount of medication can affect a lot of cells. These medications are recognized as being very potent.

But cells can also respond to less potent substances. High blood glucose is less potent than insulin, but both can affect cell behavior. Ultimately, it is the less potent substance (e.g., blood glucose) that causes the more obvious symptoms of disease (e.g., diabetes).

There is a wide range of ways that cells can communicate with each other. Since all cells depend upon each other for survival, the mistakes of a few cells can affect many others. How dangerous or helpful a substance can be is determined by the amount of substance present and its potency. A large amount of a weak substance can prove to be as dangerous as a small amount of a potent hormone.

Too much or too little of any substance can potentially affect cell behavior. Unfortunately, the amount of substance needed to cause damage can be very small.

STEP 4

The chemistry of digested food is complex and not well understood. But many patients eat an obviously bad diet. Every time we put something in our mouths, we are telling the cells of our bodies whether we want to live or not. It is food chemistry, not words, that does the talking.

If you tell your doctor that you want to live, eat like it. A pill cannot fix everything you put in your mouth. You can only feel as good as you eat...

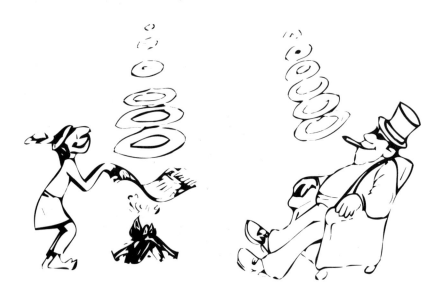

WHAT IS YOUR MOUTH SAYING?

Step 4

32. Sweet Beer, Either Way

We need fuel to live. Food gives us the fuel we need. No gas, no go.

No gas tank, couldn't go far. Without a car, we couldn't go far either. A car without a motor is a no go, even with a full tank of gas. Moving car without a driver, oh no!

S-o-o-o, fuel is not much good without the machinery that is needed to make things work. A cell is the same way. Vitamins, water, air, minerals, etc. are tools the cell needs to handle the fuel that it uses to make it go. Eventually, a malnourished cell stops working correctly, no matter how much fuel there is.

It is not possible, normally, to eat food that has fuel but no nutrients. Except for water and a few minerals, all food we eat comes from things that used to be alive. Any healthy living thing, to be alive, must have fuel, water, and nutrients (such as vitamins, proteins, and minerals). Most living things can also put extra supplies in storage.

Americans usually do not eat food that is known to have disease or that is not freshly killed, washed, etc. We do not eat road kill that the buzzards have already picked at.

The ability to consume large amounts of fuel without nutrients is entirely man-made. Everything we need to stay alive has to come from food and drink we consume. If we are missing something, chances are it is because we are not eating it when we should and could. (There are a few diseases that prevent some patients from absorbing needed nutrients.)

Alcohol is a fuel that has very little nutrients but lots of calories. Many alcoholics, skinny or fat, are malnourished. This is just one reason of many that alcoholism can be fatal.

Ever wonder what the most common cause of death is for an alcoholic? Ever wonder what there is about alcohol that kills an alcoholic? Whatever your guess is, it's probably right. That's because alcoholics die from so many things and not just from one cause. Alcoholics die, on the average, 10 to 15 years earlier than non-alcoholics. Some live a normal life span; some die much earlier. An average is just that: an average.

I'll start from the top (head).

Alcohol can fry the brain. It can cause senile dementia and seizures. One cause of dementia is well-identified vitamin deficiencies. Alcoholics are more likely to have hemorrhages (bleeds) in the brain.

Alcoholics are more likely to lose bar fights, get into severe car accidents, and be shot at. Their mouths say the wrong things while intoxicated. Speaking of mouths, cancer of the mouth, esophagus and larynx are rarely seen in nondrinkers. These cancers are very common in alcoholics who smoke.

Alcohol can poison the heart. Fatal, irregular heart beats are more common in alcoholics. Heart muscle can become so weak it can no longer circulate blood. Alcoholics can develop congestive heart failure from alcoholism. When "fluid in the lung" develops, it can rapidly turn into fatal pneumonia.

Alcoholics, when passed out drunk, can breathe in their own vomit. Vomit in the lung causes terrible pneumonia. The immune system can also be badly damaged by alcoholism, another reason for alcoholics to develop severe infections (anywhere).

Alcoholics don't always remember whom they are sleeping with. HIV is another cause of death.

Full-blown tuberculosis is not uncommon in alcoholics and can still be fatal.

Of course, there is still lung cancer...

Liver failure comes in many forms. The most famous is cirrhosis but the most common is hepatitis (yellow jaundice).

When the liver is badly damaged, options include: bleeding to death, dying from simple infections, and developing kidney failure. You cannot live without a liver.

The liver makes cholesterol. Some alcoholics develop triglycerides that are so high their blood serum looks like lard. (You can actually see the fat float in a test tube.) Gee, alcoholics die from heart attacks and strokes, too. It is rarely possible to control blood pressure in an alcoholic who drinks.

STEP 4

One of the most fatal and intractable cancers is liver cancer. Alcoholics are well represented with this cancer.

I could go on and on...

How alcohol causes all this damage is not all that well understood. We know how ice melts but we don't know why some alcoholics' brains fry.

One major fundamental problem is obvious: alcoholics have plenty of calories but are severely malnourished. Alcohol is pure energy with little to no nutrients.

Would it surprise you that drinking four cans of beer daily for forty years is not healthy? Some drink more...

Many diseases are caused by damaged, malnourished cells that are out of control (a plane without a pilot). Uncontrolled cell growth results in tumors and cancer. Uncontrolled inflammation can cause asthma, arthritis, heart attacks, strokes, colitis, etc...

Other alcoholics get sick because malnourished cells stop working. When brain cells stop working, you get stupid. When heart or liver cells stop working, you die.

Actually, beer offers a few nutrients (road kill has more). Refined caloric sweeteners offer even less. Pure energy without **any** nutrients is table sugar (sucrose).

The average American eats a pound of refined caloric sweetener every three days. That is, on average, four 12-ounce cans of soda per day. An average is just that: an average. Some drink more...

Do you really believe that four sodas per day for forty years has no ill effect?

We would condemn parents whose children drank 4 cans of beer a day. But no concern is given to 4 sodas a day. The average 6 year old child drinks more soda than milk.

This figure includes Americans who drink diet sodas. If you are not eating a cup of sugar per day, don't worry; someone else is making up the difference (by eating more). This figure includes our children. An average is just that: an average. Some kids are eating more...

Step 4

France and Russia have an epidemic of cirrhosis of the liver, because too many of their citizens drink too much alcohol. America has an epidemic, too, but ours is diabetes, because too many people drink sodas and sweet tea.

Native American Indians, before we ever showed up in this country, could not have had eating or drinking habits any further away from where they are now with today's American diet. Having never seen alcohol before the 1600s, their inability to handle alcoholism still proves fatal today. More than half of all Native American males on reservations are dead by age 18 from alcoholism.

Native Americans are also notorious for their inability to survive the current American diet. Diabetes and obesity is running rampant on Indian reservations. Record number of Indian children are obese **and** diabetic.

We are sure to follow. Like Native American Indians, we have never seen so many calories with so few nutrients before. Sugar consumption is still rising. Currently, more than half of all Americans are overweight.

If Native Americans would quit eating and drinking like Americans, they probably could get their country back in a few hundred years.

When I was a kid, my mom made me finish my vegetables, not beer or soda. Now moms want their kids to finish their "happy meals." Studies prove that fat kids make fat adults. And fat *malnourished* kids make fat *malnourished* moms who have fat *malnourished* babies...

Skinny, malnourished kids can go either way, belt-size-wise, when they grow up. But they, like skinny alcoholics, are still malnourished.

I see no difference between alcoholics and sugarholics. Both tend to die young, fat, malnourished, and for many different reasons.

Four cans of sweet beer, per day, either way, for forty years, may be more than many Americans can handle. Is that diet worth dying for?

STEP 4

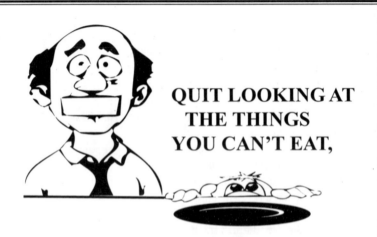

QUIT LOOKING AT THE THINGS YOU CAN'T EAT,

GO FIND THE THINGS YOU CAN EAT AND LIKE.

Most people on diets get into a rut of eating the same thing over and over again. This must be avoided so that you don't get tired of dieting. Successful dieting requires you to stop looking at old foods you cannot eat and find new foods you can eat. Once again, a calorie counter can help. In fact, you can start from the beginning of the book and go to the end, looking for low-calorie, high-fiber food items. Run your finger down two columns — calories and fiber. Stop and check out every item that meets these criteria. If it's something you like, eat it. If you don't know what it is, try it.

Review chapter 22, "*Carefully Counting with a Calorie Counter*" for more tips.

33. Finding Cause for Disease

The glory of medicine grew from the defeat of infectious disease. Scientists found the causes (bacteria and viruses) of infectious disease. This then allowed for treatments (antibiotics and vaccines) to be developed. Infectious disease as a cause of death fell dramatically. As these diseases became uncommon, expectations from physicians rose.

Today, we expect physicians to find the cause of any illness and then give treatment for cure.

For example, the most common bacterial pneumonia is caused by a "bug" named *Streptococcus pneumoniae*. This bacteria infects you; you get sick. Kill the bug; you get well. The cause of pneumonia is viewed to have originated from a bacteria. The cure is medicine, antibiotics, designed to kill the cause.

Sounds simple, doesn't it? But it isn't.

When people are exposed to this bacteria, one might get sick while many others don't. Developing pneumonia is not simply determined by exposure to a bacteria. It is also determined by the person's ability to prevent infection (immunity). Disease is the result of an interaction between two forms of life, where one develops pneumonia from the other.

The cause of pneumonia is not simply a bacteria. It's the bacteria and the patient together that create a disease we call pneumonia.

People are not the same. Our genes make us different. Our genes control our immune systems. Our immunity to the environment is also different. Some patients may have been vaccinated against pneumococcal pneumonia and are therefore more resistant to this infection. In contrast, others are more vulnerable either because of environmental factors, genetic differences, or both.

Some patients do have "bad" genes.

Bacteria are different, too. There are many strains of *Streptococcus pneumoniae*. Some have become resistant to all antibiotics. Others are vulnerable to an attack produced by our immune system. Many strains live in

Step 4

people without causing disease. Some do not.

So disease is caused by "bad genes" and "bad bugs." But more and more we see disease that does not seem to involve bacteria. For example, Diabetes Mellitus Type 2 is viewed by many as simply a genetic disorder. "It runs in families." Many people are taught to believe that genes cause diabetes.

Is it really that simple? Of course not.

There are people who easily gain weight when they overeat. Some people stay skinny no matter how much they eat. The difference is genes (if the diet and environment are the same). Therefore obesity can be viewed as a "bad gene."

However, if a famine were to occur, people who are resistant to losing weight will easily outlive those who lose weight quickly. Now the "bad gene" is good.

Dying from starvation is not considered a genetic disease. Yet, if you put 30 starving people together, none would starve to death at the same time. Some die first, others die last. One important factor for this is a person's genes that control metabolism (e.g., the rate the body uses energy).

Most people do not realize that Diabetes Mellitus Type 2 was very rare in the U.S. five generations ago. American diabetics are not some new form of genetic mutants. Instead, these patients could not tolerate overeating, the typical American diet, as well as some others.

Diabetes Type 2 became common in the U.S. because of dietary changes that have occurred over the last 5 generations. Diabetes was not caused by any significant genetic change.

Many people in poor countries starve to death; in America, we eat ourselves to death. This can be done in two ways: eat more burgers than anyone else or be more vulnerable to the hazards of burger overeating. Again, both environment and genes play a role.

Dying from starvation is no more a genetic disease than dying from diabetes. Neither disorder would hardly exist if people ate the right diet.

So-o-o-o-o, what is the cause of disease? Disease develops when our environment exceeds our genes' capacity to adapt. When our bodies can't cope, we get sick.

Medical treatment consists of environmental changes. If we are dehydrated, we get extra fluids. If we can't swallow, we put the fluid in the vein. Medication and dietary changes are other treatment options.

If we can't change the environment enough to satisfy treatment needs caused by disease, we run out of options. Eventually, genetic defects (e.g., aging) will kill us no matter what the environment is.

The relationship between life, as determined by genes, and the pressure our environment puts on us, is called "natural selection." In the wild, this is known as "survival of the fittest." In medicine, we try to lower the pressure caused by "natural selection." We do this both in treatment and in prevention of disease.

It's logical, however, that the next step for modern medicine would be the ability to change a person's genes. But to do this, we first have to understand the genetic causes of disease.

As you know, there is currently a great deal of genetic research being done. It's very likely that one day medical treatment will consist of both improving the patient's environment and the patient's genes. (This is why stem cell research may have a huge impact on treating diseases.)

But the real blow against infectious disease was not delivered by medicine. The occurrence of infectious disease that existed fell dramatically when the modern sewer system was created. Good hygiene and keeping our water supplies free of raw sewage lowered the death rate of infectious disease by 90% or more. Antibiotics and vaccines have never had the same impact.

The impact that the typical American diet has on disease will also exceed our capacity to treat disease. There is no pill that can fix what we put into our mouths. There is no gene that can cure starvation or overeating. The number one reason there is an epidemic of obesity and Diabetes Mellitus Type 2 in the United States of America is diet. The first treatment for diabetes is diet.

Eat like an American, die like an American.

S<small>TEP</small> *4*

**A PILL CAN-
NOT FIX WHAT
YOU PUT IN
YOUR MOUTH**

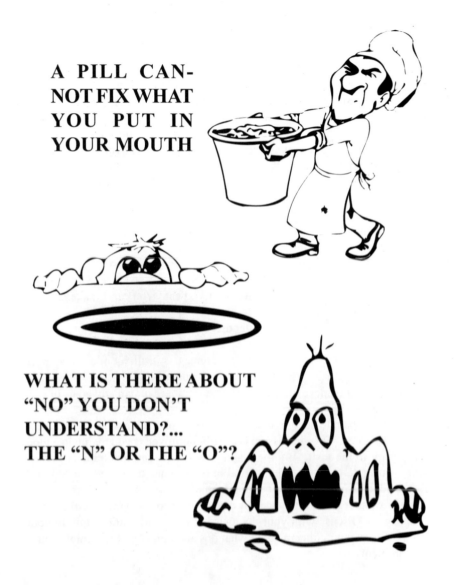

**WHAT IS THERE ABOUT
"NO" YOU DON'T
UNDERSTAND?...
THE "N" OR THE "O"?**

Step 4

34. The Do's and Don'ts of Eating

Food and water are a matter of life and death. We cannot live without food and water. It is also a matter of health. A lot of people forget that the need for a good diet applies to all of us and not just to those who are over-weight or ill. A diet is not just an issue of how much you eat or what diseases you have. A diet is not simply an issue of what weight you want to maintain.

Diet is the food that nurtures life. A good diet is about life. How well you eat and drink will always have an impact on your health and well-being. You are as good as you eat.

A good diet is defined by our goals in life. Why you eat affects what you eat. People who seek to be constipated, overweight, and suffer from excessive amounts of heartburn have different dietary goals than those who wish to avoid these problems.

Pills cannot fix all health problems. A pill is the most potent example that what you put in your mouth can affect the way you feel. So why couldn't a lot of food do the same? You are what you eat. You can't make chicken salad out of chicken crap.

For most Americans, a better diet basically means less calories, more fiber, and more variety.

Any good diet avoids dietary extremes. A little bit of a lot is better than a lot of a little. A high protein diet cannot possibly be healthy for a lifetime. Diet that does not last a lifetime cannot maintain any goals of life, for a lifetime.

Most people need to discuss with their physician what their dietary goals need to be. This discussion is greatly improved if you maintain a food diary prior to the visit. Both you and your doctor can then rapidly review what you're doing over a long period of time. The "do's" and the "don'ts" that need to be identified can be found rapidly.

Another way to enhance this discussion is to bring the lists of the next few pages. Discuss with your doctor which dos and don'ts apply to your needs. Share your concern about what dos and don'ts you feel might cause you problems.

Step 4

Improving diet is a combination of looking at what you shouldn't eat and looking for what you can eat. Most businesses have a complaint department, but not a compliment department. That is always a mistake. It's just as important to know what you are doing right as it is to know what you are doing wrong. If a lot of dietary changes are needed and identified, try to create a priority list. Rome was not built all at once but rather over time.

Progress also usually includes some steps backwards. Remember to reexamine your goals. Review which goals are being achieved and which improvements are not being made. Be sure you are aiming for the right targets. A check list is always a useful tool when trying to improve diet. Both what to do and what not to do need to be checked.

The next step to a good diet is to do it for life. You either eat to live or you live to eat. You can't do both. Practice what you preach. If you want to live, eat like it. Your doctor can only give you advice. You must accept the responsibility of making the needed changes.

For most of us, the biggest obstacle to good nutrition is not our ignorance but our unwillingness to change whatever crap (i.e. the don'ts) we like to eat to whatever good food (i.e. the do's) we should eat. You either eat because it tastes good or because it is good for you. You can't do both as the best reason. No one is perfect but mistakes do add up. Doo doos and boo boos both need to be eliminated. You are the crap you eat when you can't eliminate crap. To the best of your ability, do the do's and don't do the don'ts.

DO YOU?

A LITTLE MORE OF YOU DIES
EVERY TIME YOU CHEAT...

Step 4

Guidelines for foods to use:

Meats: choose lean meats (chicken, turkey, lamb, veal, and nonfat cuts of beef). Make sure to trim all visible fat from meat before cooking and remove the skin from poultry.

Fish: choose fish, canned fish packed in water and shellfish (lobster and shrimp should be limited to 2 per week; other shellfish can be eaten 3 times or more). Meats and fish should be broiled (pan or oven) or baked on a rack. For most people, 6 oz. of poultry, fish or lean meat is plenty. Fish is better than other white meats (e.g., chicken).

Eggs: limit the use of eggs to one a day. Eggs are high quality nutrition, therefore one per day is good, not bad. Count those used in cooking. A whole egg (e.g., yolk) is O.K.

Fruits: eat fresh fruit every day. Be sure to have at least one citrus fruit daily. Frozen or canned fruit with no added sugar or syrup may also be used, but eating fresh fruit is much better.

Vegetables: eat most vegetables freely. One dark green (string beans, spinach, or one deep yellow squash) is recommended daily (corn, lima beans etc. should be eaten sparingly since they are regarded as breads because of their starch content). Cauliflower, broccoli, celery, and potato skins are recommended for their fiber content. (Fiber is associated with cancer reduction). Avocados and olives are high in fat and calories. Eat them sparingly. The healthiest way to prepare vegetables is to steam them, but boiling, straining and braising with oil are other alternatives.

Breads: use whole grain or high fiber breads. Crackers and melba toast may also be used as bread substitutes as may pasta, rice or corn. Bread should be a good source of fiber.

Beans-Nuts: dried peas or beans may be used as a bread substitute and are a good source of protein (meat substitute). Nuts are high in fat and calories, although most of the fat is unsaturated and no cholesterol. Because most are unlikely to raise cholesterol, nuts are a good protein alternative to meat. Almonds, walnuts, and peanuts may be used sparingly (1 tablespoon), mainly for caloric reasons.

STEP 4

Guidelines for foods to avoid:

Meats, Fish: AVOID marbled beef, duck, and goose   (remove the skin from poultry), processed meats, luncheon meats (salami, bologna), frankfurters and fast food hamburgers (they are loaded with fat), organ meats (kidney, liver) and canned fish packed in oil. Less red meat, more fish and white meat (e.g., chicken). Too much of anything is not good. For example, fish is high in calories and protein (protein is low in fiber).

Eggs: limit eggs to 1-2 daily, including those used in cooking. Avoid processed eggs (e.g., egg beaters).

Fruits: avoid coconuts, which are rich in saturated fats. Avoid canned fruit with added sweeteners. Avoid dried fruit with added sweeteners. Read the labels for ingredients.

Vegetables: eat avocados and olives sparingly (when a low calorie diet is being maintained and the allowed calorie intake is so small, it may be better to avoid them). Starchy vegetables (potatoes, corn, lima beans, dried peas/beans) may be used as substitutes for a serving of bread or cereal. Watch the calories and fiber.

Bread/Grains: avoid any baked goods with shortening, white flour, and/or sugar, as well as commercial mixes with dried eggs and whole milk. Avoid sweet rolls, doughnuts, breakfast pastries (Danish) and sweetened packaged cereals Avoid biscuits. Avoid "enriched white flour"

Beans: avoid commercially baked beans with sugar and/or pork added.

Nuts: eat peanuts and walnuts sparingly. Limit all nuts as they are high in calories. Nuts are low in fiber.

Cereals: stay away from pre-sweetened cereals or cereals that list sugar as a major ingredient. Avoid cereal that has no fiber. Avoid artificial sweeteners.

Dairy Products: avoid whole milk and whole milk packaged goods, cream, ice cream, puddings made with whole milk, whole milk-yogurts and cheese, and nondairy cream substitutes. Avoid artificial sweeteners. Milk is better than soda for children.

STEP 4

Guidelines for foods to use (continued):

Cereals: choose cereals (such as oatmeal) that are high in fiber and oat bran. Read labels. To increase fiber, try mixing a very high fiber cereal (e.g., Fiber One) into any cereal you like.

Dairy Products: choose skim milk or 99% fat free milk. Also buy low fat cheese such as farmer's cheese, part skim mozzarella, ricotta or low fat cottage cheese. Use only low-fat yogurt. Some yogurts are very high in fat or sugar (calories).

Fats, Oils: use vegetable oils that are high in polyunsaturated fats (such as safflower, sunflower, soybean, corn and cottonseed). Canola and olive oil are also very good choices. Very small amounts of margarine may be used but read labels. Margarine is hydrogenated and offsets the benefit of using unsaturated oils. Many salad dressings are high in calories.

Desserts, Snacks: limit snacking. Low-fat snacks include plain air-popped popcorn, high fiber cereal without milk, vegetables (e.g., dill pickle), fruit, and any high fiber, low-calorie finger-food listed in a calorie counter. Find new things to eat.

Beverages: when you are thirsty, drink water (that's what your body needs). It is that simple. Buy bottled water if you do not like your water from the tap.

Miscellaneous: use the following freely: vinegar, spices, herbs, non-fat bouillon, and mustard. Too much of anything is bad, even "good" food. Eat, as the primary reason, because it's good for you, not because it tastes good (avoid artificial sweeteners). It is okay if it tastes good **and** it is good for you, but it is not okay if it tastes good and is not good for you.

Addendum for diabetics: eat a little of a lot rather than a lot of a little. Six small meals is not negotiable. Avoid crappy snacks. You will feel as good as you eat...but it may take six months to really feel the difference.

Step 4

Guidelines for foods to avoid (continued):

Fats/Oil: avoid butter, lard, animal fats, bacon drippings, gravies, cream sauces, and palm and coconut oils. All of these are very high in saturated fats. Examine labels on "cholesterol free" products for "hydrogenated fats." These are oils that have been hardened into solids and in the process become saturated. Margarine is one example. Avoiding margarine all together is reasonable. Salad dressings can be very high in calories (fat, oil, and sugar).

Desserts/Snacks: Avoid fried snack foods (such as potato chips) chocolate, candies, jams, jellies, syrups, and hydrogenated peanut butter. Bad, bad, bad....

Beverages: avoid sugared fruit juices, soft drinks, and cocoa made with whole milk and/or sugar. One serving of alcohol (1 oz. liquor, 3 oz. beer or 2.5 oz. dry table wine per serving) is a poor substitute for one serving of bread or cereal. If you want to improve your blood cholesterol, take a cholesterol-lowering pill (less side effects and less calories). Alcohol is high in calories, has no fiber, and not recommended.

SPECIAL NOTES:

1. Use all foods in moderation (stop eating before you feel that full).
2. Read labels carefully — sometimes they can be misleading.
3. Be sure to avoid sweets and control the amount of refined carbohydrates you eat (candies, sweets, and cakes).
4. Use a calorie counter that includes fiber.
5. Buy a good low-fat cookbook.
6. Count calories, not fat grams. Count fiber, not "sugar."
7. Eating out is usually a calorie disaster.
8. Artificial sweeteners are not nutritious, so why eat it?
9. Consult your physician if you have any questions.

35. *STEP 4* for Control of Diabetes

Diabetics who kill themselves with a bad diet do not live well. You control what you put in your mouth. You can only feel as good as you eat. You are what you eat. Today is the fourth step towards *your control* of diabetes.

Goals for STEP 4:

Review the following chapters: *22. Carefully Counting with a Calorie Counter; 28. If Losing Weight Was So Easy, There Wouldn't Be So Many Fat People; 15. Why Eat and Drink?;* and *17. Simply Read a Food Label.*

A. The following four steps should be completed:
1. Maintaining normal fasting glucose from 80 to 120 (i.e., 100+20). After meals, blood glucose less than 140.
2. Recording accurate average daily calorie count (food diary). Using food scales and measuring cup.
3. Eating more often but less (6 meals per day without gaining weight). Eat a little of a lot rather than a lot of a little.
4. No "Crap," eating more fiber (e.g., which is better — apple or apple juice?).
B. Read and review:
21. The Means and the Goal; 36. Dying to Run.; 4. Update of Diabetes Mellitus; 6. Understanding Diet for Control of Diabetes; 7. Lowering Resistance to Diabetes (only for DM type 2); and *5. Progressive Disease, Sudden Problems.*
C. Exercise plan:
1. Pick your preference. Your choice needs to be a sustained activity uninterrupted for 30 to 40 minutes. It must be done daily, rain or shine.
2. Before starting, talk to your doctor at the next office visit about your choice of exercise.
3. The likelihood of success with exercise is dependent on how practical

STEP 4

your choice is. Practicality includes: accessible daily, not done alone, not dependent on weather, and can be scheduled (morning routine usually works best).

Questions commonly asked by patients:

Do you have to be so vulgar ("crap")? Dieters tend to play-down their "little vices" (e.g., "only cheat a little bit," etc.). This attitude prevents needed change.

We are supposed to need and eat food to sustain life. Food is supposed to provide nutrients. We should eat to nurture our health. At the other end, we eliminate unwanted products (stool). Food that is bad for you is also unwanted and needs to be eliminated. Do you see the similarity? **Remember the similarity.**

In many underdeveloped countries, it is common for people to die from starvation (lack of nutrients). In America, we die from eating too much "crap." America is the fattest country in the world. "Crap" is particularly harmful to diabetics.

For a diabetic, "we are what we eat." Eating "crap" is not merely a little vice for a diabetic. Successful diabetics develop a different attitude about "crap" (e.g., high fat, high sugar, high calorie or low fiber foods). It's "no crap" — no if's, and's, or but's.

"No Crap" is simple, but very much to the point. "Crap" is not worth dying for.

Do I have to do all this "paperwork" counting calories? Yes, but that sort of thinking is a bad attitude. You cannot continue to improve and maintain your diet without writing it down. Millions of people "diet" to lose weight. Thousands maintain their dietary changes and keep the weight off. Do you complain about the "paperwork" every time you have a bowel movement? NO! The time spent doing paperwork for either end is important. Complaining about it doesn't make it easier. If you stop and think about it, it really isn't that hard to do. Whatever attitude you have about paperwork needed for your "bottom" you should keep for your top (mouth). Both eating and eliminating requires paperwork. You can either laugh about it or cry about it. Laughing is a lot more fun. Remember, only one end should handle "the crap." You choose. Your choice.

Why can't I lose more weight? If you are not achieving your weight goal, it's because you are still eating too many calories (even if it has less calories than what you ate before). We realize eating more often makes losing weight harder. But that's the way it needs to be done if you are a diabetic. Besides not taking in extra calories, you can eliminate calories by using them up. More calories can be used up faster by exercising. Exercise helps people lose weight. As a bonus, exercise also makes you healthier. Discuss your exercise plan with your doctor on your next office visit. Maintaining weight loss is more important than further weight loss. Millions of overweight people have lost weight many times. Few keep it off. Stay on the diet and weight can stay off. You will be a diabetic for the rest of your life. You will need to be on this diet for the rest of your life (if you want to live).

Why can't I eat the things I've always liked to eat? Bad attitude. Quit looking at the things you can't eat. There are plenty of new things you can find that you will enjoy. Use the calorie counter to help you find new things you can eat and like. Eat to live rather than live to eat, there's a difference.

Questions your doctor might ask you:

Can I see your food diary?
Are you finding new things to eat?
Are you eating six times a day?
Are you counting and maintaining a stable daily calorie count?
Are you using food scales and measuring cups?
Do you have any other questions or concerns?

STEP 4

IF YOU WANT TO GET OUT AND FEEL BETTER,

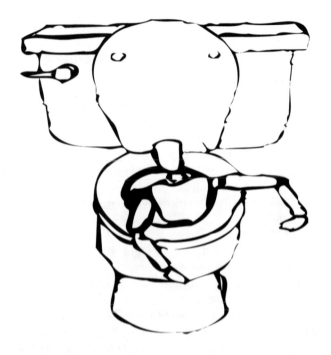

You will have to eat better.

"But the job's not done til' the paperwork's done"

Step 5

36. Dying to Run

When I was a college student, I attended a lecture on heart disease at the National Institutes of Health (NIH). The physician began with a personal anecdote as I do now. He readily described himself as a workaholic (now in recovery). He went on to tell about his massive heart attack, which forced him to stay home. He discovered that he had a "wonderful wife and family."

He realized that he needed to spend more time with his family and to reduce his workweek to normal hours. Cardiac rehabilitation encouraged him to exercise.

He discovered that running made him feel much better. So he ran. He entered his first marathon with his son and enjoyed it immensely. So he ran more. He went on to describe how much more running he was now doing. His wife and children did not run as much as he did so they fell behind.

He ran in as many marathons as possible. His doctor had recently diagnosed his leg pain as a stress fracture (broken bone) and advised him to rest. But he was going to run anyhow. He reasoned that his doctor was probably a workaholic who didn't understand the real value of running (and exercise).

At the end of the lecture, there was a time for questions. I asked the speaker if he was spending as little time with his family since he became a marathon runner as he did when he was a "workaholic." He answered that his family could spend more time with him if they would run with him since he was no longer working all the time.

I felt that he just didn't understand my question. I concluded that he went from being a "workaholic" to a "runaholic." Now crippled with a stress fracture, I wondered when he would meet the same fate as Jim Fixx, who died of a heart attack while running.

Overdoing anything is **NOT** healthy. Exercise can replace one problem with another. Fifteen years later, a more common sense and balanced view has evolved on exercise.

Exercise can be a two-edged sword. For example, exercise can either prevent or cause heart attacks. Surrounding circumstances dictate the outcome for each of us.

When the blood supply to the heart is partially blocked, exercise can easily exceed the diseased heart's ability to receive enough oxygen. Heart failure and/or sudden death can result when the heart does not get enough oxygen. In contrast, a healthy heart can be made stronger when exercised regularly. Regular heart conditioning increases body endurance, including surviving a heart attack.

As cited by my example, with time, people who exercise feel and sleep better. They have less fatigue. They feel stronger. Finally, some studies show that the size and number of blockages in the heart blood supply decrease (presumably via improved cholesterol) with exercise. All this naturally lowers your risk of a heart attack. Cardiac rehabilitation promotes exercise to aid in recovery from a heart attack (makes heart stronger) and to prevent future ones.

Running is good exercise. Walking is better exercise for those who cannot run. Swimming is kinder to feet, knees, etc., which allows for a vigorous workout without risk of stress fractures. Simply put, if you can run, running is better than walking; if you can't run (or you hate running), walking is better than running. Swimming can be the best of all if you have access to a pool.

Realistically, choose the exercise you can do. No wishful thinking.

Golf is **NOT** good exercise. Work is usually not good exercise. You must maintain a sustained increased activity for at least 40 minutes to benefit from exercise. Hard workers (e.g., construction workers) will usually work hard briefly with short pauses in between. Otherwise they couldn't last 8 hours at work. This is **not** good healthy exercise.

Find an exercise you can do year-round. Make sure you have a backup plan for hot, cold, and rainy days. Walkers can walk in the malls; runners can use home machines (e.g., treadmills, rowing machines, exercise bikes, etc.)

Good exercise can become bad exercise. A healthy leg can be made

STEP 5

stronger with running. A broken leg can be made worse with running. Injury is more likely in an unconditioned athlete (e.g., weekend warrior, ball game at picnic, etc.) Sporadic exercise is a stress test without a heart monitor or doctor. The fortunate survive. None feel better the next day.

With time, arthritis can be improved with regular exercise. Exercise can increase flexibility and strength. Initially, arthritis can be made worse, e.g., more pain and swelling. Properly done, six months later, most arthritis patients report much less pain and an increased ability to do things. They also "feel" much better. Arthritis is a reason to exercise.

Supervised exercise programs can help guide people through the right balance. Examples include fitness centers that are now a part of many area hospitals. Many of these centers have the added advantage of a year-round indoor swimming pool (great for severe arthritis).

All exercise classes help make exercise more pleasurable. Most normal people get bored exercising alone and will stop. Exercise is more likely to continue when doing it with someone else, (e.g., friends, spouse or a class).

Failure to maintain regular exercise results in rapid loss of exercise benefits. It takes six weeks to improve your body with exercise; it takes six days of bed rest to lose it. Use it or lose it!

It's easy to feel good when you are eighteen. When you are forty and want to feel younger, you have to work at it. There is no pill that can substitute for regular exercise.

If you have a chronic illness (e.g., hypertension, diabetes, arthritis, lung or heart disease, etc.), see a doctor before beginning or selecting an exercise. If you are uncertain about your current physical condition, see your doctor before starting exercise. If problems develop when you begin exercising (e.g., leg pain, chest pain, etc.), stop and see your doctor.

Properly done, regular exercise is good for you. It requires moderation and year-round maintenance regardless of the weather. If you cannot exercise on your own or you do not know how to start, supervised exercise classes are a very good idea. Staying healthy is **NOT** like running a marathon; you don't have to kill yourself to stay healthy. You can, however, ... die ... waiting.

STEP 5

AMERICAN EXERCISE

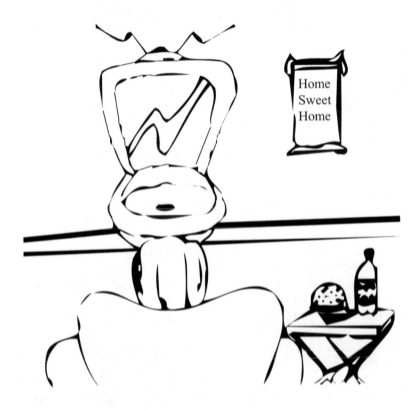

Home
Sweet
Home

Eating Crap while
watching Toilet Vision

Step 5

37. Mighty Mouth and Medicine

The mouth can have a powerful influence on our lives. Nazi Germany gave free radios to every household in the country. With Hitler's mouth, they turned an entire nation into a killing machine. I think the modern version of the old saying "the pen is mightier than the sword" should be "the mouth is mightier than a Cruise missile."

A lot of mouth in America is powered by money. Elections are won more by what is said on a radio or TV than by anything written down. Advertisers greatly influence what we do with our mouths. Beverage companies convince us to drink a lot of soda. We're so sold on sweets that the average American mouth takes in a pound of sugar every three days.

It's really amazing what a mouth can do.

If you list all the major diseases in America, you will find that they all have one thing in common. The mighty mouth determines the outcome.

There are some very impressive studies that have looked at what we can put into our mouths to help prevent disease. One of the most impressive is the Lyons study. Patients who have had either a heart attack or stroke were enrolled. All of these patients needed to improve their diet.

The Lyons study compared an "improved" American diet (dietary reduction of cholesterol, saturated fat, etc., as recommended by the American Heart Association) with one that increased fiber, fruit, vegetables which resulted in a (not-so-surprising) decline in protein, fat, etc. Additionally, patients were encouraged to eat more fish, less red meat, and use olive oil in place of butter or margarine.

The study diet is called the "Mediterranean diet." The results of the study were dramatic. Patients on the Mediterranean diet had a 50% reduction in heart attacks and stroke as compared to those on an "improved" American diet. After four years, the difference between these two groups was still widening.

It's funny how little we have heard about this study that was completed in 1998. Heart attack and stroke are the Number One killers in the USA.

Step 5

Interestingly, some patients of both groups had elevated blood cholesterol levels. At the end of the study, the number of patients with this problem had not changed. Therefore, neither diet had affected blood cholesterol.

Patients with a high blood cholesterol level on the Mediterranean diet enjoyed a decreased risk for heart attack and stroke. But these patients still had an increased risk for heart attack and stroke when compared to patients on the Mediterranean diet with a normal blood cholesterol.

Some less fortunate patients on the "improved" American diet also had high blood cholesterol level. They, too, had a higher risk for heart attack and stroke when compared to their brethren with normal blood cholesterol levels.

The conclusion was that an elevated blood cholesterol will increase a patient's risk for heart attack and stroke regardless of which diet he is on. Therefore, medication is still recommended to treat high blood cholesterol levels, even those on the healthier Mediterranean diet.

It is important to understand that the Mediterranean diet had much more impact on reducing heart attack and stroke than any change of blood cholesterol or the medication that treats it. Simply put, a pill cannot fix what you put into your mouth.

The second most deadly disease in America is cancer. Lung cancer is the most fatal cancer. Lung cancer is usually caused by the cigarettes patients put into their own mouths. The next most common fatal cancer is colon cancer (not breast). Once again, the mighty mouth plays a role.

In the past, there was confusion about whether a high fiber diet increased or decreased the chances of colon cancer. At one point, a high fiber diet was feared to cause colon cancer, but could also help the treatment of diabetes. Patients fearing both diseases would ask me what to do (diet-wise): fiber or no fiber? My answer was a question: "Which disease would you like to have?"

But now there is a general agreement that a high-fiber and/or low protein diet prevents colon cancer by at least 50% (again, by one half!!!).

STEP 5

Diabetes is our fastest growing problem. It will annoy at least one out of every five Americans. Recently, there has been a lot of press to the fact that patients at high risk to develop diabetes could prevent this disease from developing with dietary changes.

Other patients were given medication (Glucophage) instead. Those given medication also reduced their chance to develop diabetes, but their success was only half of what it was for dieters. The people who dieted were twice as likely to avoid diabetes than those who simply took a pill. Not surprisingly, the combination was even more effective.

So what were the dietary changes? More fiber, less protein, fat, and calories.

Folks, there is a pattern here. Putting excessive fat, protein and calories in your mouth without sufficient fiber (fruit and vegetables) is fatal. Excessive amounts of red meat and not enough fish adds to the trouble. Nevertheless, this is what the average American eats.

So if everything about diet is so clear, why are most of us so confused about what our diet should be? Or worse yet, why is the average American diet getting worse rather than better?

One big problem is that there is always someone who is better noticed than those that should be heard. A famous example is Dr. Atkins' diet. This high protein diet has received a great deal of publicity about how the average American can easily lose weight. Since obesity is such a big problem, the diet became a big hit. The diet has also been shown to improve blood glucose control in diabetics. This is not surprising since these diabetics are losing weight. Weight loss in diabetics, by any means, results in improved blood glucose control.

A high meat diet is basically a starvation diet composed of water and protein. That's because meat is more than 80% water and water has no calories. Protein also satisfies hunger easily. Therefore, the Atkins diet allows you to lose weight rapidly without being hungry. Since most Americans already eat too much meat, the diet can easily fit right in.

It is also well known that heart attacks and strokes are the most com-

Step 5

mon causes of death for diabetics. Therefore it would make sense for a diabetic to choose a diet that helps lose weight **and** decreases the risk of heart attack and stroke.

That is where the trouble lies. Current evidence suggests that a high protein diet will increase the chances of heart attack, stroke, and cancer. Losing weight and staying alive are not necessarily the same diet. Starving to death allows you to lose weight, but it is not a healthy, lifelong, lifestyle change.

A normal blood glucose level via weight control is not worth doubling your risk for colon cancer. Nevertheless, there are studies now being done to see if a diabetic's blood glucose control can be better maintained on the Atkins' diet. My response is, "Why bother testing this diet? A diabetic who dies from colon cancer, heart attack, stroke, etc...., with normal blood glucose, is still a dead diabetic."

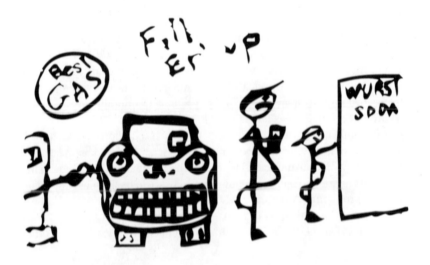

38. MOUTH MEDICINE

When we talk of "medicine" we usually think of pills (medication). We usually visit the doctor to get prescriptions for "medicine." Few think of an office visit solely for the purpose of advice. A consultation with a doctor that provides medical advice I call "mouth medicine."

The most powerful medicine for most patients is good advice that is carried out. Advice comes from the doctor's mouth. And for many diseases, the advice needed is dietary which is food and drink that goes into your mouth.

Unfortunately, despite the overwhelming, growing evidence that the most common and fatal diseases in the U.S. are caused by bad diet, most treatment plans and patient expectations are based solely on medication.

A good diet is not complicated. It's a high fiber diet with more fish, fruit, vegetables and olive oil that has fewer calories than most Americans eat. Heart attack, strokes, colon cancer, diverticulitis, constipation, obesity, gall bladder disease, and diabetes can all be treated or prevented with this diet.

So why isn't everyone on this diet? I think the medical field must accept much of the blame. Medicine is divided up into many fields and organizations. They all tend, to some degree, in the end, to be self-serving. For example, the American Heart Association (AHA) promotes its cause as the Number One problem in America. A heart attack is the most common cause of death. Amongst its membership are physicians (predominantly cardiologists) promoting their ideas about good health care.

In another field is the American Diabetic Association (ADA). It promotes its cause as the most important in America. Diabetes is the fastest growing diagnosis in America. Therefore, the treatment of diabetes is believed, by its members (including endocrinologists), to be the most important health care problem in America.

Another organization is the American Cancer Society (ACS). They consider cancer to be the worst health problem in America. Many other

Step 5

physicians feel the same way.

All of these organizations compete for the same research money and patient revenue. In other words they are competing against each other. To some degree, all of these organizations are successful.

Most women believe that breast cancer is the most common cause of death in women. That's because the ACS has successfully convinced people of this misconception.

The AHA has convinced everybody how important a low cholesterol diet is in lowering blood cholesterol (to prevent heart attacks). When diet fails (it usually does), the next recommendation is to see your doctor for a prescription. Few Americans realize how unlikely it is that diet therapy alone will lower high blood cholesterol.

Unfortunately, dietary goals that are destined to fail discourage patients from attempting any other dietary changes that may be needed. This is why I believe this misconception is harmful. All of these organizations create ad campaigns that can be as misleading as any other company trying to sell their "goods." This competitive atmosphere encourages these organizations to promote differences rather than similarities. All these organizations give dietary advice. But their advice is given in such a way that all three diets seem dramatically different. The truth is that they aren't. Nevertheless, this has left most Americans confused as to what their diet should be.

When patients are seen by a physician, they tend to get some dietary advice that relates to their diagnosis. Many patients get second opinions. Different physicians seem to give different dietary advice. The real trouble starts when patients have several diagnoses and doctors which results in a long list of dietary advice. Examples include: no salt, no sugar, no fat, no meat, no dairy products, no spicy food, no starches, no eating out, etc., etc. How about trying to choose "carbohydrates with a high glycemic index"? There are also recommendations about polysaturated fat versus unpolysaturated fat. Do you know what five grams of protein is?

Of course, there is the Web... A search produced the first twelve of a gizzilion items found.

STEP 5

Once sufficiently confused, many patients are then referred to the dietitian. Most patients quickly discover that dietitians sound an awful lot like their doctors. I don't think the confusion ends there. Then there are other sources as well...TV, relatives, etc...

Too much complex scientific advice and not enough plain answers. Most people are not sure what they should eat.

So.... what did I say, again, about the diet? It's really very simple. Eat the correct number of calories to maintain proper weight. Eat balanced meals as pictured by the USDA food pyramid in which two-thirds of your calories come from the base of the pyramid. Drink water. Eat less red meat, eat more fish and eat less meat as a whole. Boil, broil or bake your food. Olive oil should be used when cooking instead of other fats. Eat less fat. Eat much less sugar (table sugar or caloric sweeteners). Eat lots more fiber. This diet would, in fact, satisfy the concerns of most members of the ADA, AHA, and ACS. A low calorie, high fiber diet lowers your risk for heart attack, stroke, and cancer.

Both fiber and calories can be found on a food label or in a calorie counting book that lists fiber. What about salt? Put the salt shaker away and avoid processed food high in salt (junk food). What about all the other stuff on the food label? Get a Ph.D. or forget about it. Eating out? Fat chance; too many calories. Eating in? Know the cook; he or she may be killing you. Can't cook? Learn before you die. Need help? Find a doctor that practices good mouth medicine.

Yipes, that's me! (How self-serving!)

Remember that good advice isn't always what we want to hear. It's not how good it sounds that's important; it's how true it is (and that you can understand it).

Step 5

39. Fixing Links You Can Fix

Most diabetics actually die, like most other people, from heart attack and stroke. Heart attack and stroke are the Number One killers in the United States.

Doctors can calculate the likelihood (i.e. "the odds") of someone developing and dying from heart attack or stroke. These "risk factors" are well-publicized (e.g., smoking, etc.).

Diabetes is a disease where blood sugar (glucose) levels are abnormal. Diabetes is also an important risk factor for heart attacks and strokes.

So is high blood pressure, obesity, and high blood cholesterol.

A heart attack or a stroke occurs when blood flow to these areas is suddenly blocked by a blood clot. Heart cells and brain cells cannot live without oxygen or glucose. These cells are dependent on blood flow to get these essential ingredients for life.

Most people seem to readily understand that the heart and brain cannot live without oxygen. No one can normally deliberately hold their breath until they die. Obviously, our craving for air is very strong. If we hold our breath underwater, it is a matter of minutes before we must come up and get some air.

The need to breathe reflects not only the importance of oxygen, but also the fact that our bodies do not keep much oxygen in storage.

Fuel is as essential as oxygen to keep cells alive. A cell is like a tiny motor that runs on gasoline. It needs both fuel and air to run. If the fuel to the motor is cut off, the motor will stop working in less than a minute.

Our cells are the same. If the blood supply to cells lacks glucose, or if the blood supply is simply blocked, cells die in a matter of minutes.

However, unlike air, our body can store lots of fuel (e.g., fat). So can a car. Cars store fuel in gas tanks.

The ability to store fuel should not be confused with the need that fuel must be continuously supplied to the motor.

A car motor can run out of gas even when the tanks are full of fuel.

STEP 5

A broken fuel pump, carburetor, or fuel line can deny the motor the needed fuel that is in storage. Diabetic patients can run out of blood glucose in a similar manner. This is called hypoglycemia (low blood glucose levels). Hypoglycemia, like blocked blood flow, is very dangerous.

Blood vessels, like any other body part, also depend upon the rest of the body to function. The cells that form blood vessels can become diseased, especially when risk factors are present.

Diabetes, high blood pressure, high blood cholesterol, and smoking are all important risk factors that stimulate the growth of blockages in blood vessels.

Large blood vessels divide into many smaller ones. Every cell has its own very small blood vessel. These very small blood vessels are called capillaries. If a microscopic blockage occurs in a small blood vessel, only one or two cells might die. When many capillaries are blocked and cells die, noticeable disease could occur.

If a large blood vessel is blocked, a large number of cells die at one time. Obviously, the size of the blood vessel is an important risk factor as to whether a heart attack or a stroke might prove fatal.

It usually takes blockages in larger blood vessels for us to notice that we have had a heart attack or stroke.

Different diseases tend to affect different sized blood vessels. Diseases that affect big blood vessels (arteries) obviously do not have the same impact as diseases that affect many very small blood vessels (i.e. capillaries).

Diabetes is notorious for blood-circulation related problems (e.g., amputation). Some of these problems are caused solely by blockages in capillaries ("small vessel disease"). Small vessel related disease is not commonly seen in diabetic patients who only have poor high blood pressure control, but is seen if they have bad blood glucose control. Therefore, different risk factors for circulation related problems affect different blood vessels differently.

Blindness, amputation, and kidney failure typically occur in diabetics who have poor blood glucose control. Improved blood glucose control greatly reduces the chances that these problems can occur in a diabetic, even if he or

Step 5

she does not have good blood pressure control.

Heart attacks and strokes are much more likely to occur in diabetic patients who have high blood pressure or blood cholesterol (regardless of sugar control). Therefore, diabetic patients who maintain normal blood glucose control, but neglect their hypertension and/or high blood cholesterol, will probably still die prematurely from heart attack and stroke (despite avoiding the risk of blindness, amputation, and kidney failure that can be caused by diabetes). Simply having diabetes adds to the risk of heart attack and stroke even further.

In other words, treating high blood pressure will not treat diabetes (improved blood sugar control) and treating diabetes will not treat hypertension. Neglecting one risk factor will not fix the other.

The risks for heart attack and stroke do not add up as you might think. Each risk factor multiplies the increased risk for a heart attack or stroke. If diabetes doubles your chances for a stroke and having high blood pressure triples your chances for the same, the combined risk factor is 2 times 3 rather than 2 plus 3. Combining these problems with an elevated cholesterol, doubles the risk even further. This results in a twelve-fold increase for a heart attack or stroke (2 times 6 equals 12.)

Risk factors don't "add," they "multiply."

Fortunately, reducing multiple risk factors results in dividing, rather than just subtracting, these numbers.

Either low oxygen or low blood glucose is dangerous. While neglecting diabetes can prove to be fatal, neglecting other risk factors (high blood pressure, elevated cholesterol, smoking, diet, etc.) has been proven to be even more dangerous (for diabetic patients).

Life ends when the weakest link in a long chain finally breaks. Focusing on one link while neglecting another is a common, but fatal, mistake. Both air and fuel are essential. One "link" to this is good blood flow.

If it's a link you can fix,... fix it.

Step 5

HERE IS WHAT DIABETICS ARE STUCK WITH....

1. DIABETES IS LIKE A MOTOR WITHOUT A CARBURETOR...

2. THE ONLY PRICE DIABETICS PAY FOR NORMAL BLOOD GLUCOSE CONTROL IS AN INCREASED RISK FOR HYPOGLYCE-MIA.

3. SIX SMALL MEALS IS NOT NEGO-TIABLE IF DIABETICS WANT TO FEEL GOOD.

4. DIABETICS DO NOT HAVE TO PREPARE MORE MEALS, THEY JUST HAVE TO BUY MORE BAGGIES!

> **EAT A LITTLE OF A LOT RATHER THAN A LOT OF A LITTLE**

STEP 5

40. LIFELONG MONITORING CAN BE LIFE-SAVING

A little bit of knowledge can be a lot worse than no knowledge. Many people spend time and money to treat hypertension, but without realizing it, fail to achieve the desired goals. They think they are but they aren't.

The desired goal for treatment of hypertension is to stay alive and well. Merely lowering blood pressure is not (otherwise, it's just a number). It's helpful to lower blood pressure to the degree that it keeps you alive and well.

Blood pressure is measured by using two numbers. The top one is called systolic; the bottom one is called diastolic. The media has given a lot of people the impression that the bottom (diastolic) number is more important than the top. This was the prevailing medical opinion several years ago. More recent studies clearly show that the top number is more important when the bottom number is low.

Huh?

That's right. It's better to have both the top and bottom numbers a little high than to have the top number high with the bottom number too low. This predicament probably reflects the severity of "hardening of the arteries" (arteriosclerosis). The best blood pressure is when both numbers are normal.

A normal systolic blood pressure is about the same as it was when you were young (usually in the 120's). Blood pressure is never "normal" all the time. But some of the time, it should be normal. Blood pressure that is sometimes "high" is not hypertension.

The definition of "high blood" pressure (hypertension) is when blood pressure is high **all** the time, even when you are well and at rest. Since blood pressure fluctuates all the time, the best way to assess blood pressure is to check it frequently at home (not at the doctor's office). Blood pressure is normally higher at the doctor's office.

The electronic devices that read blood pressure at home can be used by most people with fairly accurate results.

Step 5

Lowering blood pressure reduces your risk for stroke much more than the risk for a heart attack. Even with aggressive treatment, the risk for either never becomes completely normal when compared with someone who has never had hypertension.

The most common causes of poor blood pressure control is forgetfulness (not taking medications as prescribed), incorrectly taking medication (miscommunication), and lack of funds (you can't take it if you don't have it). In other words, medication doesn't work if you don't take it correctly.

Factors that greatly interfere with medication effectiveness include alcohol abuse, poorly controlled diabetes, cigarette smoking, and obesity. Obesity is by far the most overlooked problem. Losing weight permanently lowers the need for treatment of hypertension. In other words, it's easier to get better results when you lose weight. Salt reduction has much less impact, long-term, on blood pressure control than weight loss.

Hypertension rarely causes sudden problems. Therefore, it is rarely an emergency to treat high blood pressure. Though rare, very sudden and severe hypertension can be a medical emergency. This occurs, more commonly, when patients on treatment run out of medication. Typical symptoms include headache, nausea, vomiting, and/or sudden visual problems. However, these symptoms are also similar to a stroke — the result of neglected, long standing hypertension (much more common).

Sudden and severe hypertension with symptoms is called a "hypertensive crisis." There are three components to hypertensive crisis: symptoms (i.e. feel sick), very high blood pressure, and there is no other cause for high blood pressure (like a broken leg).

When severe hypertension is found, without symptoms, there is no crisis. It just needs to be lowered.

Many illnesses can cause blood pressure to rise. Severely elevated blood pressure can be caused by a crisis from another illness. It is far more common that when people are not well and are found to have high blood pressure, the immediate crisis is caused by things other than hypertension.

Seeing ill patients with very high blood pressure creates a dilemma.

STEP 5

It can be very difficult to determine if hypertensive crisis is the cause or if the cause is an other illness (which came first, the chicken or the egg?). If another illness is the culprit, treating the underlying cause is much more effective than trying to lower blood pressure with "high blood pressure" medication. In some cases, lowering blood pressure with medication will make the real underlying illness even worse.

Finally, hypertension is usually a cause of impotence and not the medication. If the medication is the cause, treatment can be modified to solve this problem and treatment should not be stopped. Irreversible impotence is not the result of treatment, but rather, caused by disease (such as hypertension).

In summary, symptoms caused by hypertension take years to develop. Examples include stroke and impotence. Even severely high blood pressure rarely causes symptoms. But in some, it does and it can become a medical emergency.

When patients with poorly controlled blood pressure are not feeling well, there are usually other medical problems present. Since hypertensive patients with poorly controlled blood pressure usually feel okay, careful and frequent blood pressure monitoring is needed to ensure treatment success. Preventing strokes requires monitoring at both the home and the doctor's office.

Permanent weight reduction, by far, can give obese hypertensive patients the most lasting improvement in blood pressure control.

Hypertension usually requires lifelong treatment. When properly monitored, treatment can also be lifesaving.

41. Dead People Don't Smoke

Companies have known for years that if you can get someone to smoke for one year, you will have a customer for life. Most of tobacco marketing was based upon this fact. It's only recently that these companies have conceded to this well known fact. Get people started and nicotine would take care of the rest.

It's not surprising that tobacco marketing is targeted at young people who do not smoke. Initial exposure to cigarette smoke, for most young people, is an obstacle toward continued use. Nevertheless, many people do persist in their attempt to begin smoking. Why continue something that makes you cough, nauseated; costs money and smells badly? The answer is good marketing.

There is a lot of solid science behind good marketing. Good advertisers understand what people want and take advantage of this. Young people want to look older and be "cool." There are clever ways to satisfy this desire. For example, tobacco companies paid the original *James Bond* producers to rewrite the script so that the main character became a smoker. Now being "cool" and a smoker are associated with each other. Since children are not legally allowed to buy cigarettes, smoking is for adults.

Many young smokers persist in their attempt to smoke just as they persist to try to act older and be "cool" (peer pressure). Many successfully "persist" until they are addicted to nicotine.

Smokers are a good example of how stupid intelligent people can be and how influential advertising can be on our lives.

Smokers tend to take "cigarette breaks." For many people, smoking becomes associated with relaxation (relieves stress). Food and sex are two other common associations for smokers. Eventually, important pleasures in life become habitually associated with smoking. These pleasures in life become so strongly associated with smoking that nicotine withdrawal symptoms can be triggered when these acts occur.

Most addicts have a psychological component that can trigger physical

Step 5

symptoms of drug withdrawal and/or cravings.

What's an addiction? A craving for harmful behavior/substance that persists despite harmful effects. Withdrawal symptoms make addiction more likely but is not a requirement for addiction. Not everyone who smokes becomes an addict. But smokers who want to quit and can't are obviously addicted to cigarettes. It's not just a "bad habit" anymore. Many addicts can overcome their substance abuse when the danger exceeds the craving for the drug. Hopefully, drug use ends before irreversible harm happens.

Despite all the publicity, many smokers do not realize all the harm cigarette smoke can cause. Everyone knows about lung cancer, but the problems from smoking don't just end there. Smoking makes heartburn and high blood pressure worse. A person who continues to smoke after a heart attack has a tenfold increase to have another when compared to those who quit. Amputation, strokes and dementia are also more likely. Arthritis, asthma, and allergies are made worse with smoking. Ninety percent of black lung, brown lung, COPD (chronic obstructive pulmonary disease), and emphysema is cigarette-related. In addition to lung cancer, smoking can cause cancer of the bladder, esophagus and mouth. Cervical cancer is much more likely in women who smoke.

I am leaving out many things. This is a short list of proven facts. Smoking doesn't just make you look older. Smokers age faster and die younger. Quitting smoking really isn't a bad idea. Some smokers succeed in quitting with an all-out effort to stop "cold turkey." For those who do, great. But a lot can't.

Zyban is an antidepressant that can reduce craving for nicotine in some people. It can also treat depression and anxiety. Since smoking helps relax some people, treating unrecognized depression and/or anxiety can make it easier for these smokers to quit. Therefore, other antidepressants may be helpful for some smokers.

Smoking suppresses appetite in some people and some nicotine addicts suffering withdrawal will crave sweets. Many smokers wanting to quit are afraid of weight gain (more so than of the dangers of smoking), and in

Step 5

fact, gain weight. This problem can be prevented by implementing a low-calorie, high-fiber diet. Weight gain can also be less troublesome if smoking cessation occurs gradually.

"Quitting" gradually works well for some people. Another gradual way to prepare smokers for better success is to divide the problems associated with psychological addiction from those that are caused by nicotine addiction.

Nicotine patches can prevent nicotine withdrawal. Heavier smokers may need more than one patch per day to accomplish this. When smokers are using enough nicotine patches, persistent craving has to be more psychological in nature. The mind can crave behavior, not just drugs. Most smokers are dismayed to discover how strong psychological addiction is in influencing nicotine craving. Some smokers can't quit using patches alone.

Other smokers succeed by undergoing a gradual psychological withdrawal from cigarettes. In other words, take the "pleasure" out of smoking. My favorite trick for this is to require smokers to smoke outside. There is not much fun in having to smoke outside on a cold, rainy day. Smoking is now done solely to satisfy nicotine craving. Most smokers, over time, gradually reduce their cigarette use under these circumstances.

It is hard to quit without help. It is even harder around smokers. What are the odds of two smokers quitting at the same time? The answer is twice as bad. Make your home a "no smoking" building. Smoking outside allows one person to continue to smoke, while the other has finally stopped, without blowing smoke in their face. Both smokers will smoke less if they have to go outside to smoke.

Not all smokers succeed in quitting. I had one patient (needing an oxygen mask to breathe) who thought the hole in the oxygen mask was for his cigarette. He died smoking. I did succeed in persuading the hospital staff not to kill him for trying to blow up Intensive Care Unit.

There are a few smokers who will never be harmed by smoking. Many smokers cling to their smoking habit hoping they will be included as one of the fortunate few. However, common things occur commonly. Most

Step 5

smokers will or are paying dearly for smoking. Not only are cigarettes expensive, so is the needed medical care.

Well-trained physicians have a variety of aids to help smokers to quit. A visit to your doctor for this purpose is usually worthwhile. Smokers who want to quit, but can't, should not give up trying.

It's always easier to "try" than to succeed. But without any effort, there can never be any hope for success. When alive, it's never too late to quit smoking. It should not be a question of "if," but "when."

Dead people always quit smoking.

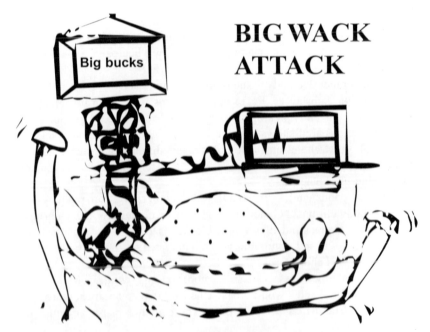

"Take out" at the ICU of Memorial Hospital

42. Suddenly It's a Heart Attack

People hear stories where a patient complained of chest pains and was thoroughly checked for heart disease. This included EKG (electrocardiogram), stress test, and/or heart catherization. Results indicated everything was okay and soon thereafter the patient suddenly died of a heart attack.

Other patients have many blockages to their heart and a great deal of angina (heart pain) but never seem to actually have a heart attack.

Why is a small aspirin, once a day, so effective in preventing heart attacks? Why is cholesterol-reducing medication (most of which is very expensive) so effective? How can stress and/or depression cause a heart attack?

Much research has been done on heart attacks, the leading cause of death in America. In the last few years, large pieces of the puzzle have been put together, giving a much clearer picture of how a heart attack occurs and how it can be prevented.

Remember that body tissue is alive — immersed in, picking up, and discarding many substances. For example, body tissues (which are immersed in blood) are constantly picking up oxygen and discarding carbon dioxide.

Heart research shows that the walls of blood vessels can pick up cholesterol, grow cholesterol-laden blockages, discard cholesterol, and/or shrink cholesterol-laden blockages. These cholesterol-laden blockages are called cholesterol plaques.

The "good" cholesterol (HDL) takes cholesterol from plaques and helps the body eliminate cholesterol. The "bad" cholesterol (LDL) brings cholesterol to plaques and allows these blockages to grow. Total cholesterol measurements will tell you nothing. Patients need to know whether they have good or bad cholesterol.

Normal blood vessels are soft, smooth, strong, but flexible. Drop or bend a rubber hose and it won't break. Cholesterol plaques are hard, rough, irregular and friable (easy to break off). These plaques cause hardening of

Step 5

the arteries (arteriosclerosis) as well as blood vessel narrowing from cholesterol plaques (atherosclerosis). Drop or bend an old, rusty metal pipe and it might break.

Inflammation can occur in response to cholesterol plaques forming on blood vessel walls. Severe inflammation can result in plaques tearing off. This results in an open, damaged blood vessel wall. Like any broken blood vessel, a blood clot can form at this site.

A heart attack occurs when a plaque tears and a big enough clot forms to block blood flow in a blood vessel supplying oxygen to the heart. Heart muscle that no longer receives a blood supply (i.e. oxygen, etc.) stops working and dies. The fancy word for heart attack is myocardial infarction (MI).

The more cholesterol plaques you have, and/or the larger the plaques are, the more likely you are to have a heart attack. The larger the cholesterol-laden blockages are, the easier it is for a small clot to stop blood flow. However, a MI will not occur if the blood clot formation doesn't occur.

Small plaques can tear, causing a lot of inflammation that forms large clots that can also block blood flow. Hence, small plaques, undetectable by medical tests, can cause an MI. A normal stress test and/or heart catherization cannot detect small plaques and cannot guarantee that a person will not have an MI.

A small MI means a small area of heart muscle has been killed. A large MI means a large area of the heart has been killed.

How quickly an MI can be recognized and treated is very important. Many heart cells do not die immediately after blood flow has stopped. New drugs (e.g., TPA, streptokinase, etc.) can sometimes dissolve blood clots and reopen blocked blood flow. The sooner this is tried, the more likely areas of heart cells can be saved. The race to save heart cells is usually won within one hour of a heart attack and lost after three hours.

Dying heart muscle can sometimes cause abnormal electric impulses which can affect the electrical system that regulates and controls heart beats (as measured by a heart monitor or EKG). Because of this danger, patients who are having or just had a heart attack are placed in intensive care units (ICU). MI patients are carefully monitored for dangerous but sometimes treatable irregular heartbeats. Once the dust settles, this danger usually passes and patients are transferred out of the ICU.

The reason low-dose aspirin is so effective in preventing heart attacks is that it reduces inflammation which could result in the tearing off of a plaque **AND** it thins blood, reducing clot formation. More is not better; high doses of aspirin are not as effective in gaining these beneficial effects.

The reason cholesterol-lowering medication is so effective is that it can stop cholesterol plaque formation. Shrinking plaques are less likely to tear. Finally, you can't tear a plaque if you don't have one.

Stress and/or depression can effect inflammation at plaque sites, affect the nervous system that controls the electrical system of the heart, cause spasms in blood vessels, may affect clotting factors, and/or cholesterol levels. In short, stress and/or depression increases your risk for a heart attack.

Current medical technology can evaluate heart vessel blockages and/or evidence of past heart attacks. Current medical technology cannot detect when future cholesterol plaques will tear or if a blood clot will form that could effectively block blood flow to the heart.

Preventing formation of cholesterol plaques is your best bet in preventing heart attacks. Opening blockages, removing blockages, and/or bypassing blockages are not nearly as effective as preventing cholesterol-laden blockages from forming.

An ounce of prevention is worth a pound of cure. This is why modern medical technology is no substitute for simple measures that begin with the patient. A patient's best bet is to lower the odds for heart disease.

Your best measures in preventing heart attacks are: regular exercise, ideal body weight, 80 mg. of aspirin (for most people) per day, normal blood pressure, high levels of HDL, and low levels of LDL. Diabetics need good glucose control and/or low insulin resistance to reduce their chances for a heart attack. Depression should be treated as this will dramatically lower the risk for heart attack in depressed patients.

Step 5

In summary, the probability of heart disease can be determined. The "odds" do not always correspond with what will actually happen. There are no guarantees in life. One can only increase or decrease the odds. But no matter what the odds, it can suddenly be a heart attack.

HONEYMOON is OVER

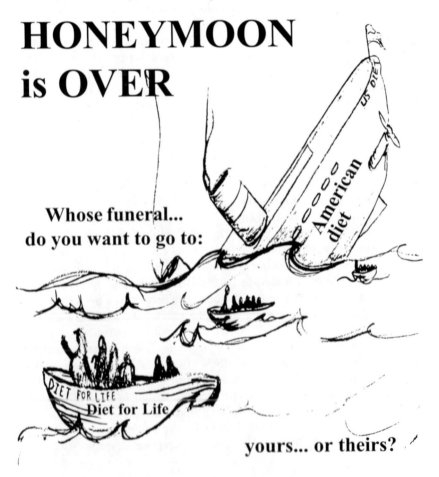

Whose funeral...
do you want to go to:

yours... or theirs?

Step 5

43. The Gospel on Cholesterol

Remember when salt was "bad"? Researchers observed that blood pressure could be lowered when hypertensive patients reduced salt intake. The press forgot to tell us that high blood pressure returned — for most people — once the body adjusted to a low-salt diet.

The "healthy heart crusaders" had struck again. Nevertheless, bad press wiped out salt as a preservative in the food industry.

Now, fifteen years later, we know that patients who suffer from congestive heart failure and/or renal failure need to watch salt intake. However, for most people high salt intake means more trips to the bathroom.

The number one verse sung by the "healthy heart crusaders" for many years was (and still is) that dietary cholesterol influences the risk for heart disease. Simply put, more dietary cholesterol, more cholesterol in the blood, more heart attacks (MIs). Better safe than sorry; eat less cholesterol and blood cholesterol will go down. Very simply put... but not very true.

It's been rough for egg farmers the last 25 years. For the record, an egg is one of the cheapest, "natural," high-quality protein, multivitamin, high-mineral snack for the buck. The only problem with eggs for some people is that they eat too many. Weight-watchers, beware; too many eggs have too many calories (but one does not). One per day is usually enough.

Healthy heart crusaders forgot to tell us that the body can make cholesterol from scratch. Therefore, the body can determine a person's blood cholesterol level without any dietary cholesterol input. While in a few patients blood cholesterol will fall with a low-cholesterol diet (no harm trying), most patients' blood results will show little to no change. I have observed this for years as a physician. Ironically, a strictly vegetarian diet (zero cholesterol) can make blood levels of cholesterol go up in some patients. (Huh?)

Recently the healthy heart crusaders are starting to admit that dietary changes can change blood cholesterol by no more than 6% on average (which isn't much). Therefore, dietary changes for the sole purpose of lowering cholesterol yield very little results (one big exception, diabetics with poor

Step 5

sugar control).

So what is and what is not important about cholesterol?

Cholesterol blood levels — regardless of how the level was achieved — are important. But total cholesterol is not. Huh?

Most cholesterol panels have two parts — good and bad. The higher the LDL (bad cholesterol), the higher the risk for heart attack or stroke. The higher the level of HDL (good cholesterol), the **lower** the risk for heart attack. Vice versa — very low HDL (regardless of the LDL level) is an independent increased risk factor for heart attack.

So! A person with high total cholesterol due mostly to **very high** HDL has a very low risk for heart attack. A person with **low total** cholesterol due to very low HDL has an increased risk for heart attack. See why a total cholesterol number does not tell you anything?

It's been fashionable for people to get free — or cheap — total cholesterol screenings. This is a waste of time and money. You need a Lipid panel with a breakdown on the different kinds of cholesterol before you can assess a person's cholesterol for risk of heart disease.

An even more complicated breakdown of the cholesterol profile will become increasingly more available. In this panel, total LDL can be broken down into even smaller parts and HDL likewise. Some of these parts will be good and some will be bad.

Cholesterol panels include calculations that magnify slight differences in measured lab results (including lab errors). Therefore, several Lipid panels over several months should be checked before concluding how good or bad your overall cholesterol profile is.

What makes cholesterol profiles good or bad? Number one on the "bad" list is poorly controlled diabetes via failure to comply with your diet. Number one on the "good" list is increasing HDL via exercise. High triglycerides lower HDL (which is bad). But we don't know much else about triglycerides — like, for example, why they are high. For that matter, we don't know, in many people, why the cholesterol panel is bad or good. Genes certainly play a role. So did diet when you were a baby. Babies who are fed

Step 5

breast milk (which is incredibly high in cholesterol and fats) tend to have better cholesterol panels as adults.

Huh?

The cholesterol profile mirrors your risk for heart attack or stroke — with incredible one-for-one accuracy. Over and over again, it has been proven that the high risk cholesterol profile patient is more likely to suffer heart attack or stroke. The higher your risk from additional factors (e.g., diabetes) for a heart attack, the more important your cholesterol panel becomes. Adults do not need excessive fat or cholesterol. No one denies that. Yet, as newborn babies, it seems we do. Breast milk is very high in fat. So when does this dietary transition occur? What and when should children be eating less fat to improve their future adulthood cholesterol panels? Answer: we don't know. One dietary change we can definitely recommend: eliminate sugar (e.g., sodas, candy, etc.).

How can bad results from a blood cholesterol panel be improved (treated)? This is easy.

Regardless of why the cholesterol is bad, cholesterol-lowering medication can improve it. It's not the "natural" way to do it, but the medicine sure does work. The resulting improved cholesterol panel gives (and this has been proven) lower risk for heart attacks and/or strokes (As before, these improvements correspond one-on-one). The lower, the better.

The safest, easiest-to-take, effective drugs are expensive — approximately $80+ a month (hearts of gold!). Poor folks can try cheaper, older drugs but most cannot tolerate the side effects. But even with medication, wealthy diabetics and/or obese people still need to be on a diet (and exercise).

Television ads for cholesterol-lowering medications make mention of "liver problems." This is not a serious problem. How many people do you know who died from liver failure compared to those who died from a heart attack or stroke? A simple blood test can be done to make sure everything is okay. Indeed, blood tests need to be done anyhow to follow your cholesterol profile after treatment begins.

Step 5

Finally, proper exercise is helpful. But don't forget the author and famous advocate for jogging, James Fixx (author of the *Complete Book of Running, 1977*). He died of a heart attack while jogging 20+ miles a day. He did this knowing that he had a terrible cholesterol panel. The lesson here is that not everyone's cholesterol will respond to the "healthy heart crusaders' gospel," Verse 2: *exercise*. Jim Fixx should have taken medication to lower his cholesterol. He did not — a lethal mistake. A heart deprived of a decent blood supply does not get stronger or healthier when exercised. It's simply at risk of failing (from lack of oxygen) as it tries to meet increased demands from exercise.

In other words, if a bad cholesterol panel does not improve with exercise, then you need to stop. Before resuming exercise, fix the blood supply (lower your cholesterol) to the heart. Don't forget you need to fast at least 12 hours (*OUCH!*), so a blood cholesterol panel can be drawn from your vein when you come in for your doctor visit. **WHEW!**

> **Normal blood glucose (sugar) control is for the diabetic who is sick and tired of being sick and tired**

Step 5

44. Deadly Mix and More Pills

The average patient with hypertension (high blood pressure) is on three to six drugs. But the average patient doesn't end there. Many hypertensive patients have other medical problems that require treatment (pills). Worse yet, these other problems usually increase the concern hypertensive patients already have — a higher risk for heart attack, stroke, and kidney failure (dialysis).

For example, an elevated blood cholesterol will dramatically increase your risk for heart attack or stroke. While a low fat, low cholesterol diet is touted as an important way to improve blood cholesterol, most patients will only achieve recommended goals with medication. (A rather expensive pill, I might add.) This also means that the average hypertensive patient is on four to seven drugs when you include the treatment for cholesterol.

A much more deadly combination for a patient with hypertension is obesity, diabetes and elevated cholesterol. The addition of three more risk factors is not additive (e.g., $3 + 3 = 6$ fold increase in risk). Rather, these risk factors multiply the increased odds for heart attack, stroke or kidney failure (e.g., $3 \times 3 = 9$ fold increase in risk). For those who know mathematics, the increased risk goes up exponentially when risk factors are summed up.

Unfortunately, overweight diabetics are likely to develop hypertension and have high cholesterol. Vice versa, obese patients with early hypertension are more likely to develop diabetes, etc. This deadly combination of risk factors is becoming increasingly more common in the United States as more Americans become overweight. This combination can result in the doubling of recommended medications needed for treatment.

So what's your reaction to a patient taking a large number of pills (a bag full)?

I thought so.

Let's look at it from the other side. If "normal" persons increase their chances of a heart attack because they have high blood pressure by 10%, being a diabetic triples that chance. Medication that treats these prob-

Step 5

lems lowers risk factors by division, not subtraction. It's not minus 3; it's a risk factor that is lowered by a third. Sooooo, if you were a diabetic patient with a tremendously increased risk for heart attack, stroke or kidney failure, would you pass up the opportunity to cut that risk factor by one-third? Multiple risk factors require multiple medications (a bag full of pills). I have never seen a doctor become distraught when a patient stops taking a whole bag of medication. I have, however, seen many depressed patients after an amputation, stroke, or heart attack. It's the patient, not the doctor, who suffers the consequences of untreated hypertension, etc. Most patients, at least in hindsight, prefer taking their medication.

There are instances where patients receive too many medications. Doctors sometimes prescribe too much medication. Sometimes patients demand too much medication. The needs for medication can change and there can be a failure to recognize the need to reduce or stop medication. However, there are many "bags full of medicine" that are properly prescribed. Patients with multiple risk factors require multiple medications to reduce those risk factors.

If you are one of those patients with a "bag full of medicine" and you are considering stopping one or more of these drugs, discuss this with your doctor before you make those changes. Doctors do not always make it clear to patients why they are on medication. The indicated uses found on labels and in books may not be the reason you are taking that medication. It's wise to know the possible consequences of your decision before you make that decision.

The cost of a full bag of medication is enormous. Patients with many medical problems can easily spend much more money at the drug store than for rent or mortgage. For elderly patients, these costs can exceed the entire Social Security check. Taking twelve pills a day may sound unbelievable, but it happens a lot more than you realize.

It's also worth noting that once a patient develops any of the aforementioned disorders (hypertension, diabetes, elevated cholesterol) before retirement, getting life or health insurance becomes almost impossible. Natu-

STEP 5

rally, it's the people who need health and life insurance who cannot get it. If you are ever curious how high your risk factor is for heart attack or stroke, just apply for insurance. If you get rejected outright, or your premiums are much higher than normal, then you know that your risk for heart attack or stroke is high. Though you can improve those odds at any time, your ability to acquire insurance will probably never change.

So how can America solve this problem? Well, one way is prevention. The average American can avoid this common medical nightmare by improving his/her diet. In other words, don't eat like an American (and then you might not die like one). It also helps if you exercise (as opposed to the average American).

Many of my patients have regrets when they look back on how they took care of themselves over the years. Some damage done can be repaired, but some cannot.

There is bad luck and there is dumb luck...

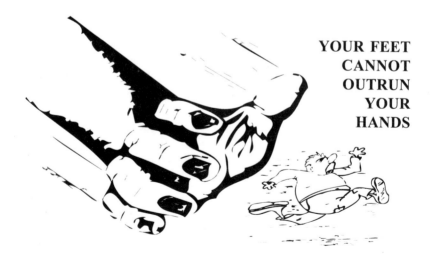

YOUR FEET CANNOT OUTRUN YOUR HANDS

45. Goals for *STEP 5*

If you're not part of the solution, you're part of the problem. You have two choices: grow old or die young. Today is the fifth step towards *your control* of diabetes.

A. Before starting exercise:
See your doctor.
Consider a stress test.
Have your feet checked.

B. You and your doctor have agreed on the following goals:
1) Normal Glucose: maintaining fasting glucose from 80 to 120 (i.e. 100+20), after meals <140.
2) Calories per Day (six meals per day):_____
3) Target Weight (if losing weight, <3 lbs. per week):_____
4) Daily Exercise (>30 minutes per day):
      What? _____
      Where? _____
      When? _____
      Any Help? _____

C. Record Daily Weights in Food/Glucose Diary. Weigh yourself on the same scales at the same time every day. Even if the scales are not accurate, almost all scales will accurately weigh differences in weight (this is our primary interest). We suggest weighing yourself first thing in the morning without clothes. Adjust calories as directed by *22. Carefully Counting with a Calorie Counter* to obtain weight goals. If exercise-related problems develop (e.g., chest pain) — **STOP** and call or see your doctor.

Questions commonly asked by patients:

STEP 5

Who said life is fair? No one should say that. When you are a diabetic, you can't eat like you once did. It takes six months or longer to become fit with diet and exercise, but it only takes six days to lose the progress you've made (weight control and/or physical fitness). Small mistakes can cause big problems. It may take years for high glucose to kill you, but it only takes ten minutes for low glucose (hypoglycemia) to do the same. The price you pay for maintaining normal blood glucose as a diabetic is that it is easier to get hypoglycemia. In the long run, it's a price worth paying. It's easy to feel good when you are young. You have to work at it when you're older. It's worth it. Quality and quantity of life improves.

Does exercise make arthritis worse or better? Initially exercise can make it feel worse. That's why you need to start your exercise gradually. Properly done, exercise will eventually make arthritis feel better. In six months time, your arthritis will probably feel the best it has in years. Physical therapy, cardiac rehabilitation, and professionally instructed exercise classes can help you properly start and maintain your exercise program (however, these things are not always necessary).

How can I find the time and energy to exercise? How many times during the first four steps for your control of diabetes did you say that you couldn't do half the things that you are doing now? If there's a will, there's a way. There are twenty-four hours in a day. Thirty minutes represents two percent of that time. Exercise can improve your energy levels and your ability to sleep better. Exercise is one of the few things you can do that will reverse the damage caused by diabetes (e.g., heart disease). It also makes it easier to lose weight and control sugar. Your body works better once you are more physically fit (use it or lose it). You can do more when you feel good.

Getting there is the tough part. If you want to feel good, you must work at it. Exercise and diet.

If I work hard all day, why should I have to exercise? To survive an 8-hour work day, hard work is not maintained continuously. In addition to any breaks, many small pauses are needed and included in the work day. This

Step 5

prevents exhaustion and allows hard work to continue. Exercise to improve physical fitness requires increased activity that increases both breathing and heart rate **uninterrupted** for at least thirty minutes. Exercise cannot last eight hours and work cannot substitute for exercise. Hard work (increased activity) can help lose weight (burn calories).

Can't you control my glucose with medication (just pills!) without diet and exercise? As we have said many times, temporarily, yes. In the long run, **no.** Review previous chapters if you don't remember the reasons why. All the building blocks for your body come from food. In the long run, you are what you eat.

Questions your doctor might ask you:

Do you want to live?
What goals (glucose, calories, target weight, and exercise) don't you understand?
Do you have any symptoms of heart problems?
Have you had any symptoms of hypoglycemia?
How do you treat and prevent hypoglycemia?
How do you handle unplanned events that interfere with planned meals?
Are you having any problems with glucose, diet, weight, or exercise?
Do you know all your medication bottles?
Are you finding new things to eat?
Are you eating six times a day?

Step 6

46. Keeping Diabetic Feet

Unfortunately, amputations are not uncommon for diabetics. Understanding how and why amputations become necessary is helpful in understanding how to prevent these kinds of losses.

Our shoes wear out and are replaced regularly. Our feet repeatedly outlive our shoes. Shoes are not "living" but our feet are. Can we conclude that our feet are indestructible? Of course not!

The fact is, we simply don't see that our feet do wear. The small but continuous loss of tissue is replaced by new tissue growth. The survival of our feet depends on the body's ability to replace damaged and destroyed cells with new cells. Replacement tissue needs to arrive at the same rate as tissue is destroyed in order to keep the status quo.

This precise process takes place every time we take a step. Feet are not indestructible. Most people fix their feet as fast as they tear them apart.

The forces our feet survive daily are tremendous. When walking, our entire body weight rests briefly on areas the size of a dime. Forces increase even more if we jump or run.

Preventing damage to our feet requires the ability to feel forces that are becoming harmful. We call this "pain." Stepping on a nail instead of a dime exceeds the skin's ability to support our body weight without piercing the skin. Pain protects. Pain makes us move the foot away from the nail (as soon as possible).

Hopefully, the pain reflex will prevent the nail from piercing the skin. If harm does occur, pain discourages us from striking the same area again. This allows time for healing (which is new growth).

The longest nerve fibers in the body extend from the brain to the feet. The longer the blood supply, the more places problems can occur anywhere along its length. Therefore, the longer the nerve, the easier it is damaged and eventually harmed by poor blood supply (i.e. high blood glucose levels). The death of thousands of long nerve fibers eventually leads to no feeling in the feet. The fancy medical word for this problem is polyneuropathy.

Step 6

Feet without feeling can be harmed without detection. Harmful blows and excessive pressure result in destruction of tissue. This can easily reoccur when there is no sensation to warn of the danger.

Tissue destroyed from excessive trauma can exceed the healing capacity of the foot. Furthermore, the healing capacity itself is damaged by the same factors that harmed the sensation of the foot in the first place (more factors to follow).

Cholesterol blockages in blood vessels are not uncommon in diabetics. When these blockages are in the heart's blood vessels they cause heart attacks. Other blockages can result in stroke. Complete blockages in leg blood vessels result in death of that part of the foot or leg.

Sufficient constant pressure applied outside of a blood vessel will crimp the vessel, stopping blood flow as well. Once blood flow stops, the body's areas dependent on that blood supply can die from lack of oxygen.

Anyone can briefly sit on one's own leg. Later, that leg "falls asleep." This occurs because the person's weight puts enough pressure outside the blood vessels and pinches them closed. Cells stop working when there is not enough blood. But the pain and discomfort (pain protects) remind us to get off of our leg so blood flow can be restored. Failure to do so would result in irreversible damage to the leg. This is likely to occur if there were no sensation in our legs to warn us of this danger.

Leaking fluids anywhere in the body fall downward. The feet are usually the lowest part of our bodies. This leakage would naturally collect in our feet. Excessive fluid in tissue causes pressure that results in swelling. Again, pressure outside the blood vessel can stop blood flow. Therefore, excessive fluid causing feet to swell creates pressure outside the blood vessels in the leg. This creates a poor blood supply to that area.

Returning blood back to the heart can be a problem for the feet. Blood pumped by the heart **down** to the feet has to somehow be forced back **up** to the heart. (In contrast, blood pumped **up** to the brain can simply fall **down** to the heart.) The one-way valves in the veins needed to do this task can fail (e.g., varicose veins). Blood not successfully returned to the heart pools in the legs, causing swelling. Worse still, blood cells in this pooled blood die there. These ruptured cells cause inflammation which causes more swelling.

It doesn't stop there for some patients. To make matters worse, many diabetics have had bypass surgery in which veins from the legs had to be removed. This, too, causes an incompetent venous system.

Swollen feet from any cause damages the tissue of the feet. This damage includes the nerve endings under the skin's surface. Once these nerve endings are destroyed, sensation is lost. Loss of sensation is an invitation for more insult and injury to the feet.

All these problems feed on each other. It's not surprising that diabetic feet can die. Everything we've described is a vicious cycle. Loss sensation increases destruction of tissue and increases swelling. Swelling impairs blood flow and, without adequate blood flow, tissue repairs poorly and more nerve endings are destroyed.

If any part dies, and it cannot be replaced, gangrene sets in. Most gangrene rots off. The hole it leaves behind becomes a source of infection and body fluid loss. Either problem can be life-threatening.

Sometimes dry gangrene sets in. Instead of rotting off, these dead parts become "preserved." Examples of dry, dead tissue are the well-preserved mummies found in Egypt. This process is not very different from cow skin being turned into leather. Unfortunately, like shoes, dead body parts eventually wear off and, once again, a hole is formed. It's difficult and dangerous to ignore gangrene.

Saving feet involves many strategies. Foremost of these is to preserve the ability to feel (i.e. slow or stop the damage to the nerves and nerve endings). Pain protects. This means swelling in our feet needs to be reduced and blood glucose (sugar) needs to be controlled (kept normal).

The causes of feet swelling are mechanical (e.g., gravity, broken vein valves, surgery, etc., etc.). The solution is mechanical as well: compression stockings (very tight socks) extending to just below the knee are by far the most practical solution for swollen feet. A tight stocking squeezes the fluid

Step 6

out of the foot and up the leg. Standing on your head is more effective but not nearly as practical. However, when possible, keep your feet elevated as well (preferably above your heart).

Contrary to popular belief, diuretics (water pills) are **not** an effective solution to leg swelling. There are exceptions to this rule.

Good footwear can protect numb feet from harm. Don't walk barefoot. What constitutes "good footwear" is discussed in another chapter "*Feet physics and good footwear.*"

Finally, if you can't feel your feet, that doesn't mean you can't see them. Careful visual inspection for damage, such as broken skin (cuts) or calluses, needs to be done daily. Early discovery of damage should initiate damage control (treatment). Diabetics with damaged feet need to see their doctor immediately.

The bottom of the foot (most difficult to see) is the area that requires the best inspection. A mirror or a second observer is best. *There can be no shortcuts in this daily exercise.* Shortchanging the quality of the inspection results in bigger defects to be found at a later date. The bigger the area affected, the more likely gangrene can occur and amputation will be required.

Neglect makes many diabetic problems worse. Diabetics who protect their feet prevent or delay amputations. Delays in amputation result in more years of walking.

It's that simple.

If you are a diabetic at any stage, see your doctor on a regular basis. In order to keep your feet, you must learn what needs to be done. Then do it.

MODIFIED USDA
Food Guide Pyramid
A Guide to Daily Food Choices

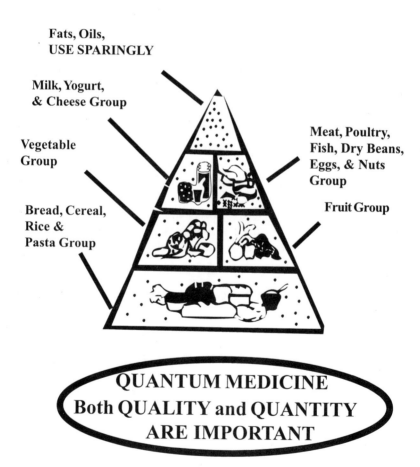

**Fats, Oils,
USE SPARINGLY**

**Milk, Yogurt,
& Cheese Group**

**Vegetable
Group**

**Meat, Poultry,
Fish, Dry Beans,
Eggs, & Nuts
Group**

**Bread, Cereal,
Rice &
Pasta Group**

Fruit Group

**QUANTUM MEDICINE
Both QUALITY and QUANTITY
ARE IMPORTANT**

STEP 6

47. PREVENTING FOOT PROBLEMS FROM DIABETES

Carefully wash your feet every day using mild soap and water. Do not use hot water. Dry your feet gently, particularly in between your toes. Pat your feet dry, rather than rub them dry.

Check your feet closely before putting shoes on and immediately after removing them. If you cannot see, find someone who can. Look between your toes and over the soles for any blisters, cuts, scratches, cracks, thick corns, or new growths. Any problem like this justifies a visit to your doctor as soon as possible. When in doubt, check it out, ASAP! (Remember, trying doesn't count.)

Each day apply a mild moisturizing cream after you have washed your feet to prevent dryness and cracking. Do not put cream in between the toes. Do not walk barefoot after applying cream.

Change your socks/stockings daily. Cotton socks with absorbent layers are best. Before putting on your shoes, make sure that your socks are wrinkle-free. Replace any socks that have tears or severe wear.

Do not go barefoot. Your shoes should fit well. Slippers and slip-on shoes are not well-fitted shoes. Choose shoes that are laced, well ventilated (e.g., leather), well-fitted, have insulated soles, and are free of defects. Avoid shoes with pointed toes. Good shoes do not squeeze your toes. Instead, the shoe should match the shape of your foot.

Do not wear the same pair of shoes for more than two days in a row. This helps prevent wet feet that can cause foot sores. Know how to cut toenails properly (not too long, not too short). If you nick your toe, see your doctor. Your doctor may need to refer you to a podiatrist. You may need to see a podiatrist on a regular basis (ask your doctor).

Step 6

48. Polyneuropathy: Battle Lines Drawn for Feet

It's bad enough to have any disease. To add insult to injury, disease can cause other diseases. It is not surprising that problems can develop when the body's blood supply (that every cell depends on) isn't quite right.

Any bad blood supply can cause polyneuropathy. Alcoholism, smoking, vitamin deficiencies, rheumatoid arthritis, hypertension, etc., etc., can all cause this problem. Diabetes is one of the worst and most common cause of polyneuropathy. S-o-o-o-o, what's "polyneuropathy"? It is a disease that is difficult to explain. S-o-o-o-o, why bother? Because the most common form of polyneuropathy is the biggest reason most diabetics lose their feet (amputation).

For some people, "nerves" refer to a nervous or mental condition (psychiatric). But nerves can also refer to multiple "wires" that leave the brain, form the spinal cord, and are then distributed throughout the body. These nerves transmit and receive information between the body and the brain. A nerve is like a telegraph wire that carries Morse code. The signal is either on or off (beep or no beep). With nerves, the meaning of the signal is determined by source, location, and the frequency of the signal. Knowing the source and location of the nerve gives the same kind of information as color-coded wires and electrical/technical manuals (used by repairmen) do.

An activated nerve ending for pain from your toe sends the signal up the nerve where it arrives at the brain. The brain, knowing where the nerve originated, along with the intensity of the signal and the function of the nerve (different nerves do different things), figures out your foot has been hurt. The brain converts this signal into the feeling and/or the concept of pain (toe pain, to be precise).

Simply put — no brain, no pain.

Pain is always in your head. It is an idea that is usually triggered by stimulated nerve endings. Without thought, there is no pain. "I think, therefore I am" (*Descartes*).

Other nerves (wires) send down commands from the brain to cause

Step 6

muscle movement, etc.

A nerve can be damaged anywhere along its length. An injured nerve can be stimulated (by the injury) to send signals to the brain. The brain usually concludes that the signal originates from the nerve ending rather than anywhere along its length. These mistakes are called "referred pain." A good example of referred pain is the "funny bone" in your elbow. When the elbow is struck in a certain way, the blow strikes a bundle of nerves which go down your arm. This blow causes sharp electrical pain to shoot down to your fingers. It feels as though your hand has received an electrical shock, despite the fact that the origin of the pain is a blow at the elbow (which the bundle of nerves crosses).

Nerve cells can also be killed. Dead cells stop working and no more signals can be generated. Depending on their function, patients either experience loss of sensation (i.e. numbness) or paralysis.

However, for some people, the brain can decide it still feels something even though the nerve ending isn't there, was not stimulated and/or is dead (i.e. not functioning). A common example of this is an amputated leg. Patients can commonly feel a limb that is not there. Phantom leg pain is a form of referred pain.

Unlike other cells (such as skin which can grow back), nerve cells cannot be replaced when killed. For both brain cells and nerves, cell death is irreversible and permanent.

The longer the nerve, the more likely the "wire" can be cut or damaged. Compare this to an army at war that is dependent on long supply lines. When under attack on many sides, long supply lines are more vulnerable to being weakened or cut off. The most advanced positions of troops are the most susceptible to losing needed supplies.

Nerves in the body depend on a blood supply to stay alive and function properly. For most people, the longest nerves are the ones that go from your head to your feet. These long nerves also have the longest supply lines.

When supplies are cut off, not all problems are immediate. Soldiers carry some supplies with them that must be used up before they "run out of ammunition." Nerve cells do the same. Eventually a soldier or nerve can no longer function and will die without supplies.

While a soldier low on supplies can continue to function, he is usually more vulnerable to injury or death. Likewise, nerves under attack and low on supplies are vulnerable to cell death.

Diabetes Mellitus is a disease that affects the fuel supply of every cell in the body. A cell cannot function properly without the correct amount of fuel and oxygen (just like a motor). The longest supply lines are, naturally, the most vulnerable to the damage caused by high blood sugar (diabetes). The longest supply lines have the smallest reserves and are the quickest to run out of fuel when blood glucose is low. Therefore, poorly controlled blood sugar in diabetics disproportionately harms the longest nerves in the body first.

How and where body cells are killed is important. Other diseases, like stroke, attack a cluster of nerve cells that are clumped together.

Similarly, the effects of casualties on a battlefield also differ by how and where they occur. One small area of a front can be completely overrun and wiped out. This same number of casualties has a different impact on a battle if these losses were to occur throughout the line (or ranks). The number of soldiers wounded, rather than killed outright, also affects the battle outcome. All this is also true when cells in the body are attacked by disease (e.g., diabetes).

Wounded soldiers initially tend to demand more attention than actual dead soldiers. Conscious, wounded soldiers yell (sometimes still fight). Dead ones don't. However, dead soldiers will eventually have more impact on the outcome of battle.

As cruel as this sounds, a single casualty or wounded soldier rarely has any significant effect on an entire army's performance. Large numbers of dead and/or wounded are always more noticeable than smaller numbers. Our bodies are made up of many cells. The loss of a few cells is rarely noticed. Many damaged/dead cells are.

Polyneuropathy is the medical word for "disease of many nerves."

Step 6

"Poly" means many. "Neuro" refers to nerves and "pathy," to disease. When many nerves are injured or killed, after being attacked by disease, this condition is called "polyneuropathy." The longest nerves are the ones most affected by diseases that cause polyneuropathy. The severity of the problem is determined by the number of nerves affected, the severity of the wounds (i.e. how badly nerve cells are damaged), and causalities (i.e. nerve cells killed).

Wounded or damaged nerve cells, by their injury, are stimulated and triggering pain (usually a tingling or an electric shock sensation). Painful, damaged nerve cells cause even more pain when the nerve endings are also stimulated (e.g., touched). Initially, cells causing pain are much more noticeable than cells that have already died (and are without feeling). Eventually, it's the dead ones that add up.

Diabetics experience this pain as burning or tingling of the feet that is made worse by light touch (e.g., putting socks on). Although their feet may feel like they are on fire (tingle, "fell asleep," etc., etc.), the fire is not there. Instead, this is referred pain from many damaged nerves (polyneuropathy!).

Severe pain indicates a lot of nerve cells are wounded. Severity of injury and the number of cells that die occur gradually. If this pain is replaced by numbness, it may be that many wounded nerve cells have finally died. Relief from the pain of polyneuropathy by numbness is an indication that damage from disease has gotten worse, not better.

A foot without sensation is like a soldier without eyes and ears. A numb foot becomes extremely vulnerable to lethal injury. Once gangrene sets in, the foot must be amputated. This is not uncommon when diabetes (i.e. blood glucose control and diet) is neglected. Most wounded soldiers, if neglected, will also die. Civil War battles were notorious for this. At the end of every battle, fields were littered with wounded men crying for help. Little was done for them so most died. Many of these casualties were preventable even with the medical knowledge of the time.

Pain is good in that it lets you know that something is wrong. Untreated, the end result of polyneuropathy is that the feet become completely numb. Neglected, wounded nerve cells die.

Step 6

Treatment for pain caused by polyneuropathy is also needed. Treating the underlying cause does not necessarily get rid of all the pain or damage all ready done (it does stop or slow down the progression of polyneuropathy).

Pain control options include antidepressants or medications used to treat seizures. Nerve cells are made up of the same stuff as brain cells. It makes sense that medications which can affect the brain can also affect the nerves themselves. In this case, reduce the pain.

In my opinion, traditional pain medication (such as narcotics and arthritis medicine) is neither very effective nor helpful with referred pain (e.g., polyneuropathy). Referred pain is a different kind of pain than that which is triggered solely by nerve endings (the pain does not behave in the same way). Different treatment... for different pain.

The use of antidepressants or seizure drugs does not make referred pain less "real." Remember, all pain is in your head. No brain, no pain.

Pain from polyneuropathy is a pain that should not be ignored. Pain isn't all bad; severe numbness is. A foot without sensation can step on a piece of glass and the brain is never told. A foot without sensation cannot detect blood loss, cuts, infection, etc., etc ....

A foot unprotected by the warning signals of pain (sensation) can be damaged faster than the body can heal. When the destruction of a foot exceeds the body's ability to heal, the foot is lost. Unfortunately, for the diabetic, sensation is not the only thing damaged by poor blood glucose control. So is the ability of the body to heal.

Every time a diabetic cheats on diet or glucose control, another nerve cell (or cells) is attacked, wounded or killed. A good food supply for a diabetic is a matter of life and death. While individual losses can go unnoticed, the casualties of battle can only add up. The number of dead never decreases. Dead nerve cells cannot be replaced. So many diabetics "cheat" on their diets that many people fail to recognize how important diet and blood glucose control is. Diabetics who have always maintained their diets and blood glucose control rarely develope polyneuropathy. The others commonly do.

Step 6

The ultimate treatment for polyneuropathy is prevention. When polyneuropathy is diagnosed, the underlying cause should also be determined. If at all possible, these problems need to be treated. For a diabetic, that means good blood glucose control and diet.

The battle to keep feet will be lost if the supply line against polyneuropathy is not improved. Which do you like better? .... feet or food? If you are a diabetic, one depends upon the other.

What happens

when the slo-o-o-w-est gun
has the biggest mouth?

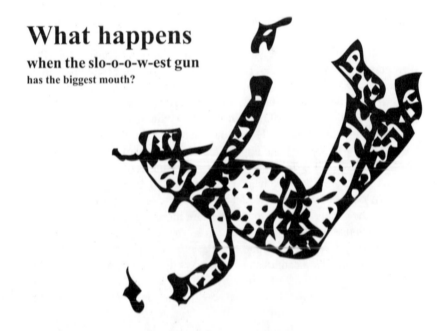

49. Feet Physics and Good Footwear

When my ex-wife went shoe shopping, "comfort was the key" to her final selection. (I wished prices were.) For those who cannot feel their feet (such as some diabetics), shoe selection is not so easy. Without feeling, comfort cannot be well judged. Improperly-fitted footwear can result in unnecessary amputation. To understand what is needed in a "good" shoe, it's best to understand what goes wrong with a "bad" shoe.

Your hands have never taken the beating your feet have. Feet take a terrible pounding. The forces involved are much greater than you might think. Math and physics illustrate this well. I'll try to keep the math simple (e.g., the only way you can be sure you get the correct change for a purchase is by doing the math). In the world of science, mathematics can sometimes dramatically illustrate important points. Some people don't like math. Nevertheless, if you want to understand some ideas, you will have to work through the math.

In America, pressure is measured in pounds per square inch (PSI). Weight is measured in pounds. The area to which this weight applies force to is measured in inches. The size of a square (or rectangle) is measured on two sides (length and width). Multiplying these two sides will give you the area (the space inside the box) of the square. Hence: pounds per square inch.

I weigh 240 pounds. I stand on two feet. Each foot is twelve inches long (my foot **IS** a foot!) and approximately two inches wide. The area of one foot (2" X 12") is 24 square inches. Standing on two feet doubles the area (24 + 24 = 48 square inches). My weight (240 lbs.) divided by the area (48 sq. in.) which I stand on (two feet) gives a pressure of 5 PSI. If I stand on one foot, the area is halved and the pressure increases to 10 PSI.

Suppose instead that I try to stand on one big toe (tiptoe) of one foot? Having tried, I have found that the pressure on my big toe becomes very uncomfortable. I cannot stand that way (tiptoe) for long. Two hundred forty pounds standing on a 1/2 inch by 1/2 inch area (0.25 sq. in.) increases the pressure to 960 PSI. In contrast, car tires are inflated to 30 to 40 PSI.

STEP 6

Your car owner's manual can provide you with the recommended tire pressure. No one drives a car with tire pressure greater than 100 PSI. Inflating a tire to 960 PSI would provide quite an explosion.

The math shows us that the pressure applied to the foot is greatly influenced by the size of the area that bears the weight. The smaller the area, the worse (i.e. higher) the PSI. It should be clear to you why having a pebble in my shoe hurts. If my foot stands on a small pebble (e.g., 1/4 in. X 1/4 in.), a pressure of 3,840 PSI is felt at that spot. *OUCH!* Most pressure washers operate in the range of 1,600-3,200 PSI. A pressure washer is powerful enough to blast water through cement. Can you now imagine the destructive forces of 3,840 PSI?

Pain protects. The pressure exerted by the pebble creates pain. I stop bearing weight on this area because it hurts. I find the pebble before I resume standing on that area. Patients who lose sensation in their feet cannot feel pain. Instead, they continue to walk on the pebble, unaware of its presence. The pebble easily has the opportunity to puncture skin and damage the foot. To make matters worse, the math of physics states that force (**Energy**) is the summation of one half the **Mass** (weight) times the **Velocity** (speed) squared (multiplied). A physicist would write $E = 1/2\ MV^2$ (huh?). In plain English, a baseball bat hits harder (energy) if you swing it (velocity) *and* it is heavy (mass). Walking on a pebble hurts more than standing on one. The impact of walking on the feet is greater than that of the standing body weight. Running (increased velocity) increases the forces even more. *Now* do you understand what your feet must endure!

"Good" footwear helps protect feet against these kinds of pressures and forces. If your shoes perfectly match all the contours of the bottom of your feet, PSI falls and comfort increases..

A cement floor cannot adapt to the contours of bare feet. The success of firm padding that is not too soft inside your shoe is based on its ability to form the exact shape of your foot (increasing the weight-bearing surface area of the foot). The outside of the bottom of the shoe has to be hard enough to support huge amounts of weight on a small area (high PSI). These

Step 6

high pressures can be lowered by transferring the same weight to the inside of the shoe over a large surface area. This weight transfer carried out by shoes is what protects your foot against a pebble laying on the ground outside your shoe. One final point about footwear: you cannot fit a square peg into a round hole. The shape of your shoes should be the same as your feet. If not, a small area of your foot will press against the side of your shoe that doesn't match your foot. The smaller this area, the higher the PSI. Here we go again...

Custom-made shoes for medical purposes (numb feet) are very expensive (up to $600). Materials used date back to the treatment of leprosy. Lepers lose body parts because of loss of sensation. Materials were developed for these patients that could fit and adapt precisely to the contours of feet (in all directions). This material greatly reduces pressure on completely numb areas, preventing gangrene, and can delay loss of limbs.

For diabetics, good footwear prevents or delays amputation. Amputation costs thousands of dollars to perform. Prolonged nursing care and physical rehabilitation add to the cost. Finally and eventually, an artificial leg must be made (they cost *more* than $600). Good footwear is so important in saving money (Medicare doesn't necessarily care about limbs) that Medicare has actually started to pay for custom-made shoes for diabetics. Only diabetics on insulin who have foot problems qualify. Other insurance policies vary as to their willingness to help patients with numb feet keep their legs.

Good footwear can save money and disability (suffering). Before buying custom-made shoes, see your doctor for evaluation of your condition and needs. Not everyone will benefit from custom-made shoes, so good (comfortable) shoes from the store may suffice.

Where there is Medicare money, there are con-artists. Be sure the person or company making and fitting your shoes is competent and honest. Your doctor may know someone he can recommend.

Unfortunately, not all numb feet can be saved. A variety of other factors can cause gangrene and amputations as well. However, for those

STEP 6

feet that have lost the ability to feel pain (sensation), good footwear still adds up to be a limb-saver.

If sensation in your feet is declining (feet tingle and burn), see your doctor. If your feet are numb and any foot problem has developed, see your doctor. You would be surprised how often foot surgery can be avoided if foot problems are handled properly and on time. Better late than never does not always apply to your feet.

MODERN U.S. JET FIGHTERS ARE ARMED WITH SOME OF THE MOST LETHAL WEAPONS WE HAVE EVER CREATED...

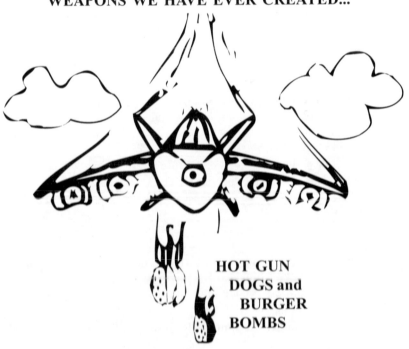

HOT GUN DOGS and BURGER BOMBS

Step 6

50. Goals for *STEP 6*

You will always feel better and do better with normal blood glucose. Diabetes is not worth dying for. The only price a diabetic pays for having normal blood sugars (glucose) is an increased risk of hypoglycemia. Today is the sixth step towards *your control* of diabetes.

You need fuel to go. Your energy depends on how you eat. If you eat too many calories, you either gain weight (fat is stored calories) or your blood sugar becomes too high (flood the carburetor). If you don't eat calories when needed, you run out of gas. Calories count. Count calories. It is important to have energy and it's worthwhile staying well.

Reread (review!): 6. *Understanding Diet for Control of Diabetes,* 22. *Carefully Counting with a Calorie Counter,* 21. *The Means and the Goal,* and 36. *Dying to Run.*

Goals for STEP 6:

A. You and your doctor have agreed on the following goals:
1) Normal Glucose: Maintaining fasting glucose from 80 to 120 (i.e., 100+20), after meals <140.
2) Calories per Day (six meals per day):_____
3) Target Weight (if losing weight, <3 lbs. per week):_____
4) Daily Exercise (>30 minutes per day):
       What? _____
       Where? _____
       When? _____
       Any Help? _____
B. Avoiding avoidable hypoglycemia. Frequent small meals. Eat more often but less. No skipped meals. No late meals. Eat on time using the correct number of calories. Meals with (increased) fiber do much better in preventing hypoglycemia.
C. The same, the same, the same... Daily routine helps control blood

STEP 6

glucose. Regular routine helps control diabetes. *Same* bedtime, *same* wake-up time, *same* calorie count (*same* energy in on time), *same* activity level (*same* energy out on time), the same, the same, the same, etc, etc..... To maintain normal glucose, you have to match the same calories with the same level of activity, every day, at the same time.

D. Different Food, Different Food, Different Food ... You cannot eat the same food every day. Balanced meals require all the different food groups. You do want to eat the same daily calories. Adding fiber whenever possible is also very important. Eat a variety of quality food (more fish, less meat). This means no crap. No ifs, ands, or buts.

Questions commonly asked by patients:

How can you expect me to do everything the same? It is not easy, but remember that routine helps control glucose. With careful planning, there are diabetics who have traveled around the world with perfectly normal blood glucose. If there is a will, there is a way. The kind of activity does not have to be the same, but the amount of exertion (i.e. effort or energy used) needs to be approximately the same every day. This includes weekends. Food doesn't have to be the same, only calories per meal need to be the same (and at the same time). "Energy in" cannot match "energy out" without a plan (schedule).

Why do you keep making the diet harder? Because diabetes gets worse, not better. As you get older, unfortunately, there are many things that get worse. Diabetes is just one of those things. Falling apart (with age) won't stop, you can only slow it down. Eventually, your sugar control will become harder to maintain. More medicine will be needed and added. Sooooo.. to keep your diabetes under control, your diet cannot stay the same. It has to keep getting better. Do this before you lose control over your sugar.

Aren't there always exceptions to a rule? No, not always. Skipped meals cause life-threatening hypoglycemia that can kill you. As diabetes becomes worse, sugar control becomes more difficult to maintain. It is also easier to develop hypoglycemia. To prevent this, "energy in" needs to match "energy out." Routine activity prevents skipped meals. Meals on time (at the same time) with the same calories (that have worked in the past) will work in the future. The same, the same, the same....prevents hypoglycemia.

Why is my sugar so high after hypoglycemia? The body knows hypoglycemia is dangerous. The body has all kinds of ways to try to raise blood sugar when it is too low. Usually, when desperately needed, the body succeeds in raising blood glucose (usually too much). If not, you die. Therefore, hypoglycemia can cause high glucose. High sugar can also cause low sugar. Poorly controlled diabetes can be a "yo-yo" of sugar control (keeps going up and down). This is why diabetics who have poor ("yo-yo") sugar control always feel bad. They also tend to die much younger. Frequent meals with fiber and the right number of calories—on time—is your best protection against hypoglycemia.

Do I have to keep eating different things? Yes! Because the quality of food, not just the quantity, is important. You are not just eating calories, you are eating nutrients. It is very important that a diabetic has a nutritious diet. When you eat less, it is a lot easier to not eat enough of any needed vitamin, mineral, protein, etc., etc.... Eating many different things helps ensure a balanced and nutritious diet. The purpose of diet is not simply to provide the correct amount of energy or calories. Your diet should be designed to sustain and nurture life while it keeps your blood glucose normal. Quantity & Quality.

Eat a little of a lot rather than a lot of a little.

Questions your doctor might ask you:

Did you bring your food diary (counting calories)?
What was your sugar (blood glucose) on _____*? (any day of the week)*
What new foods have you tried?
Are you eating more vegetables, more fruit, more fiber, less meat, and no crap?

STEP 6

Are you getting better at eating on time?
What goals don't you understand?
Do you know all your medication bottles?
Do you have any questions or concerns?

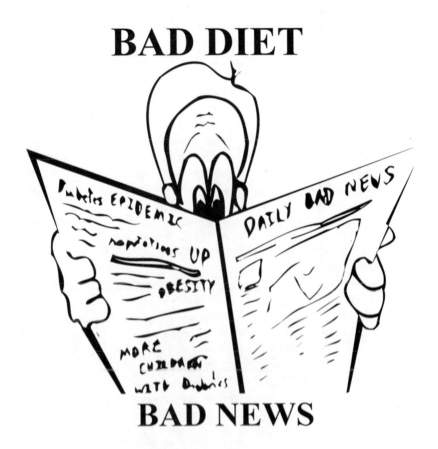

Step 7

51. Preventing More than Heart Attacks

The human body is composed of many different living cells. All of these cells came from one cell that was fertilized by one sperm. As the fertilized egg grows and creates new cells, some of these new cells begin to specialize in form and function. Specialized cells of one kind form different organs, e.g., heart, lung, or brain. It's easy to forget the incredible miracle that the entire human body came from one cell.

All of our cells become dependent upon each other to survive. For example, all of our cells need oxygen. We obtain oxygen by using muscle cells to breathe in. Our lung cells are organized to put oxygen into red blood cells. Our heart cells are synchronized to contract in such a way as to pump blood throughout the body. Through a complicated system of blood vessels, every cell in our body receives oxygen. It's also easy to forget that the heart must pump blood and oxygen to itself as well. Heart muscle cells need oxygen and some of the blood flow passing through the heart must come back around to the heart itself to supply the heart's oxygen needs. Even the lungs need a blood supply to provide oxygen. Not all lung cells are exposed to air.

Cells without oxygen (no blood supply) die. When heart muscle is deprived of blood, we call this a heart attack. When blood flow to the brain is blocked, we have a stroke. When the blood supply to a leg stops, the leg dies and an amputation is required.

For most blood vessel blockages, the cause is the same. Blood vessel walls develop a disease called atherosclerosis. These blood vessel walls develop areas filled with cholesterol, called plaques, that grow and fill in the opening of the blood vessel. Eventually, some plaques rupture and become inflamed. The result can be a blood clot which can completely block blood flow.

An alternative to blocked blood flow is the rupture of the blood vessel. Cholesterol plaques can weaken the blood vessel wall. The pressure inside the blood vessel expands the weakened wall like an overinflated bal-

Understanding **DIABETES**
IN BLACK AND WHITE

TEN STEPS TO CONTROL DIABETES

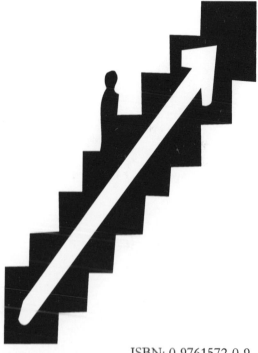

ISBN: 0-9761572-0-9

By **Mark E. Meijer, MD**
Board Certified Family Physician

TEN STEPS TO CONTROL DIABETES

Learn from a Board Certified Family Physician who taught patients how to help themselves. For more than 10 years Dr. Meijer has created Patient Education handouts using words ordinary people can understand (no medical gobbledygook). Unusual humor is added that helps keep diabetic patients and their families motivated to control this disease at their own pace.

1. His readable book educates people step by step,

2. His slogans and mnemonics create aversions towards a bad diet,

3. His strategies lead to a permanent and successful lifestyle change.

TREATING DIABETES THROUGH DIET IN A REALISTIC MANNER

Dr. Meijer's Diabetes Management Program (MDMP)© persuades and teaches diabetic patients and their families how to control Diabetes. This is done by emphasizing dietary goals and not just relying on drugs or shots (or even surgery!). Changing the usual "normal" American diet (high calorie and low fiber) to a healthy one (low calorie and high fiber) is a ten step program.

Step 7

loon. This "balloon" is called an aneurysm. As aneurysms grow, they become easier and easier to rupture.

The end result of a ruptured aneurism is similar to a blocked one: no blood flow. Blood leaves the artery instead of traveling downstream to its planned destination. Once again, organs are deprived of oxygen.

Formation of plaques filled with cholesterol must be stopped in order to prevent strokes, heart attacks, aneurysms (bleeding to death), and many amputations. Things that promote plaque formation should be avoided.

The simplest plaque former to avoid is cigarette smoke. Stop smoking. The exact ingredients in cigarette smoke that promote plaque formation are unknown. Lower tar and nicotine cigarettes are not less likely to form cholesterol plaques. So much for "safer" cigarettes.

Elevated cholesterol levels (of certain types) increase plaque formation. There is a direct relationship between cholesterol levels and cholesterol plaque formation. This makes sense and studies have repeatedly shown the importance of reducing cholesterol levels in order to reduce anyone's risk for a heart attack or stroke.

However, most people forget that the body can make all the cholesterol it wants even if we don't eat cholesterol. For many people, diet does not change blood cholesterol levels since the body, not the stomach, determines those levels. Regardless of the cause of increased blood cholesterol, lowered levels will reduce plaque formation. In some cases, these plaques will shrink.

Medications designed to lower cholesterol are very effective in reducing cholesterol and preventing all diseases caused by plaque formation.

High blood pressure increases plaque formation and lowering blood pressure decreases formation of cholesterol plaques. It's not entirely clear how lowering blood pressure helps prevent plaque formation; nevertheless, it does regardless of how the blood pressure is lowered.

There is, however, one class of blood pressure medication that directly acts on stopping plaque formation. This class is called ACE inhibitors. Examples include Vasotec, Univasc, Lotension, Capoten, Accupril, etc.

STEP 7

Another approach to preventing heart attacks and strokes is to simply remove the cholesterol plaque. When these blockages exist in blood vessels supplying the heart, balloon catherization can be done. Another trick for this problem is to build vessels that bypass the blockage. This is called "bypass surgery." When blockages exist in the neck arteries to the brain, these can be removed, also, by a procedure called endartectomy.

Finally, when aneurysms are found, these can be fixed with artificial grafts.

America does more surgery on blood vessels than any other country in the world. Unfortunately, surgery does not stop new plaque formation nor can it fix more than a few locations. Therefore the surgeon only addresses the biggest and most obvious blockages caused by cholesterol plaque formation.

Unfortunately, there are many blood vessels everywhere throughout the body. All these blood vessels came from a single source. Where there is one blockage, there will be other vessels affected the same way.

Preventing heart attacks, the number one killer in the U.S.A., prevents all kinds of other medical problems. Heart attacks and strokes are the most notorious problems but many other areas can be affected as well. Many other common medical complaints can be attributed to poor blood flow. Hearing loss and impotence are two of many examples.

Here's my point: one heart attack represents only one blockage among many. Any patient who survives a heart attack is at risk for another from other blockages. Furthermore, that patient is also at risk for a stroke, aneurysm, amputation, etc., etc.

It cannot be emphasized enough how important it is to prevent cholesterol plaque formation. Doing so prevents problems throughout the body. Plaque formation is a systemic problem throughout the body. Surgery alone is very limited in saving lives

Controlling blood glucose, not smoking, losing weight if overweight, increasing exercise, controlling hypertension, lowering elevated blood cholesterol levels, eating more fruits, eating more vegetables, eating more whole

Step 7

grain breads, eating more fish, and eating less fat and/or refined sugar (eating less, period) helps prevent cholesterol plaque formation....

WHEW,... that can get to be a long list!   It can be an even longer list of medication...

Simply put, eat like an American, die like an American.

The old adage "an ounce of prevention is worth a pound of cure" really applies here.

52. Why Now?

Life hangs in the balance. Status quo is usually taken for granted. Adverse change creates problems and solutions seem more apparent if the cause of the change is known.

Diagnose, then treat.

Simple problems, such as catching a cold, seem straightforward. We become infected by a virus, we get sick, we fight infection, and then we get better.

But why now?

Viruses are everywhere. Why get sick today and not yesterday or tomorrow? Did our immune system weaken or did we get exposed to an unusual number of virus particles? What other factors could be involved? No one really knows.

A person with a cold can be in a room filled with well people. Some of them will get sick and some will not. All receive (presumably) approximately the same exposure.

Contrary to popular belief, there is no evidence that "we catch a cold" (infection) just because we got wet on a cold day. Colds are caused by viruses. Viruses don't care how wet or cold we are.

The real question is why we don't get sick *every* time we are exposed to a virus.

Some people go for years without being sick only to have one year where they have frequent colds. Later, they become well again and for years, again, remain well. The "bad" year, in many instances, cannot be explained. All tests done during that time come back normal.

No matter how hard surgeons try, a small number of patients develop wound infections. In most instances, the "cause" can be grown by the laboratory and identified. However, these same bacteria can also be found in patients without obvious wound infections.

For most patients, the straw that "broke the camel's back" is not apparent.

Step 7

There are circumstances where it is blatantly obvious why we become sick. It's easy to understand why an AIDS patient with a dying immune system gets infections. It's also obvious why people exposed to huge numbers of bacteria or viruses also get sick. What's not clear is why some of us get sick on some days and not on other days.

Medicine can statistically predict how many people will get sick within a population. But on an individual basis we do not know who will stay well and who will actually become sick. Predicting treatment results are the same. Two patients can have the same cancer; one responds to radiation and the other does not.

Flipping a coin behaves in the same way. Statistically, we can predict the odds of heads or tails (50-50). What we cannot do is predict when each head or tail actually will occur.

Preceding events do not affect future odds. However unlikely, a million heads in a row do not change the odds for the next coin flip; the odds are still 50-50.

Statistics are used to calculate the "odds" of many important events. These statistics were created from past experience and good record-keeping. Doctors take this information to calculate odds for diagnosis or prognosis. Prognosis is the forecast of how an illness will behave.

It is understandable that patients with terminal illnesses (or their families) become concerned about time. "How long?" Predicting a death is based on statistics of previous patients with the "same" (i.e. similar) illness. From this data (i.e. past experience), probability of life expectancy can be determined. Predicting precisely how long anyone can live can **not** be determined. I can tell you what the odds are but I can not tell you the day and time.

I'm faced with this question "How long?" all the time. I give patients or families two choices: I can be very precise and completely wrong **OR** I can be completely right but totally imprecise.

Precise time can be measured in years, months, weeks, days, hours, seconds, one-tenth of a second, one-one-hundreth of a second, etc., etc.,

etc.... The odds that a patient will die at precisely the given moment predicted by me or anyone else is practically zero. The odds are much more likely that the patient will either die before or after that time and date. Even if I tried to shoot the patient near the time of predicted death, I could not cause death at such a precise moment.

In contrast, I can be completely right in predicting time of death if I am allowed a very safe margin of error. The weather forecasters do this all the time. I can predict with total certainty that a patient will die between 0 and 200 years from now. Unfortunately, this prediction is as good as no prediction at all.

Medicine is filled with possibilities and probabilities. No physician can be 100% right. Even if the physician were always right in stating probabilities, this still wouldn't give patients precise outcome. This is why, in medicine, there are no guarantees.

No matter what the odds are, eventually the patient faces the events that actually do occur. Once this event has occurred, the prediction (diagnosis or prognosis) becomes irrelevant.

For example, if the odds are a million to one that you could die from Medication "A" and you do, the odds of survival become irrelevant (no matter how good they were).

Cause and effect can also be confused with statistical coincidences (technically called correlation). If two things occur commonly then it is possible for both of these things to occur near each other. Furthermore, there can be a pattern that one tends to precede the other. Nevertheless, this does not prove that one causes the other.

I have had patients who were very fearful of insulin. All the friends or relatives they knew who began insulin then subsequently required an amputation. This pattern convinced them that insulin caused amputations.

The fact remains that both problems are caused by diabetes. As time progresses the need for insulin use becomes increasingly more likely. Usually later still, amputation also became increasingly likely as the diabetes progresses.

STEP 7

But insulin **DID NOT** cause the amputation. In fact, with diabetes, neither can occur, one can occur, or one can occur without the other. Statistically, the most *probable* scenario is that one will follow the other. Common things occur commonly.

Statistical probabilities do not prove cause and effect. The mysterious straws that "broke the camel's back" can be multiple and/or very small. In many instances, cause can not be determined since the straws are too small to be seen by current medical technology.

As important as "cause" can be in understanding disease and in helping to find a cure, many illnesses begin without any reasonable explanation. Patients with difficult medical problems that cannot be adequately treated become very frustrated trying to find "a cause." "Why me? Why now?"

My answer is, "Only God knows." Based on statistics, medicine's answer is "Why not?"

Step 7

53. Living Longer, Hearing Less

It's easy to take for granted what we already have. Losing something (especially unexpectedly) is a painful reminder of what we have had (and taken for granted). Suppose you were given a choice of which to lose, would you choose sight or hearing?

Most people choose and think deafness is preferable to blindness. In truth, the opposite is better.

Imagine going to a family dinner or on a date where you cannot hear a word. Try to satisfy a customer or a boss that you cannot hear! Life without a phone or a radio. Loss of hearing affects social contacts dramatically. Losing hearing is a lonely business.

The importance of sight is paraphrased by the old adage "do not judge a book by its cover." Ultimately, human relationships are not built by how people look; instead they are built by words (most easily spoken and heard). While intimate relationships can be built by letters sent far away, most people will find that their relationships are an "earshot" away.

You can hear neither the rain nor an ambulance siren. It's hard to stay in tune with the world from day to day or from minute to minute if you cannot hear anything. Losing sight does not isolate people in this way.

Most people know that hearing loss occurs with age, especially after long exposure to loud noises or shorter exposure to even louder noises (such as cannons). What is not commonly known is that hearing loss associated with aging is a peculiar problem of modern civilization (i.e. the Western world). Deafness with age does not exist in the jungle (i.e. undeveloped countries).

Scientists have found primitive tribes in the jungle that face lifelong exposure to loud noises. For example, some tribes live next to large and loud waterfalls. Measuring this noise, scientists found that these tribes were exposed to noises much louder than those that the average city dweller hears. Despite this, elderly tribesmen hear very well. There was no tendency among these people to lose hearing with age.

Age and noise were not a risk factor for hearing loss in the jungle. In fact, deafness was extremely rare.

Reexamining the statistical analyses showed that other risk factors were needed to explain hearing loss in this country. This additional risk factor was vascular disease in any form. In other words, all the same risk factors for heart attacks and strokes, the leading cause of death in the U.S.A., contribute to hearing loss. These factors include obesity, Western diet, cigarette smoking, elevated cholesterol, elevated blood pressure, diabetes, and a sedentary lifestyle.

Scientists have concluded that the damage needed to cause hearing loss had to come from both sides: loud noise from the outside and poor blood supply from the inside.

For many, ringing in the ears (called tinnitus) is the first sign of hearing loss. This is usually a sign of high frequency hearing loss, which usually occurs first. Therefore, most hearing loss associated with age is not a uniform and total loss. Lower frequency sounds can still be heard well.

Unfortunately, important parts of communication (the spoken word) require the ability to hear high frequencies. The ability to hear speech deteriorates faster than hearing loss as a whole, making the spoken word increasingly more difficult to understand. This loss prompts most people to seek help (i.e. hearing aids).

Hearing aids amplify sound. The sound of speech can be better heard with a hearing aid. Unfortunately, the magnification of sound does not usually match hearing loss. Some frequencies, which can be heard well, are inappropriately amplified. Hearing aids can make these frequencies sound too loud.

While hearing aids make higher frequency sounds audible, they also make other (usually lower) frequency sounds uncomfortably loud. The sound of a spoon falling to the floor (low frequency sound) becomes painfully loud (as loud as a cannon). It is commonly known that loud noises make hearing loss worse.

Hearing aids can be expensive.

Newer hearing aids can selectively amplify frequencies to match hearing loss. Newer and more expensive. Small ones are also easy, but expensive, to lose. Matching hearing aid perfectly with hearing loss can be difficult to maintain even when achieved. People, including their ears, can change.

Hearing aids become a kind of "damned if you do, damned if you don't" device. Some patients tell me hearing aids can sometimes be a pain in the ear... (who teaches patients to talk that way?).

Ironically, cataracts are also not seen in the jungle. This problem is also associated with the Western world (civilization). However, in contrast to hearing treatments, cataract surgery is very effective and curative. Therefore, as we age, going deaf **and** blind is not usually necessary.

The best treatment for hearing loss is prevention. Avoid unnecessary and excessive sound. Some jobs do require hearing protection. Some don't. Either way, protect your hearing by avoiding excessive noise (e.g., ear plugs). Hearing can also be protected by designing environments that produce less noise. At home, mufflers need to be replaced promptly and stereos can be turned down. All this makes for better retirement years.

Modern medicine, despite the way we take care of ourselves, manages to keep us alive longer, more than ever before. Ironically, this also puts us at even more risk for losing our hearing. The longer we live, the more likely it is that we will lose our hearing.

The need to prevent heart attacks and strokes in America is great. This not only saves lives but preserves the quality of life as well. No matter how hard we try, medical care can never replace preventive care (e.g., no smoking, healthy diet, and exercise).

Every year, graduating seniors celebrate with a senior dance or prom. The music at these events is so loud you can actually *feel* the music. Graduation does more than mark the next step in these young people's lives; it also marks the point where hearing loss seems to begin.

Autopsies of dead American soldiers of recent wars (young men in their teens) show extensive evidence of early heart disease. In contrast, soldiers of undeveloped countries show no evidence of heart disease.

History tends to repeat itself. The next generation of Americans seems determined to do as we have done before: smoke, overeat, not enough exercise, and too much noise.

    Monkey see, monkey do. Hear no evil? No. No *hear* at all!

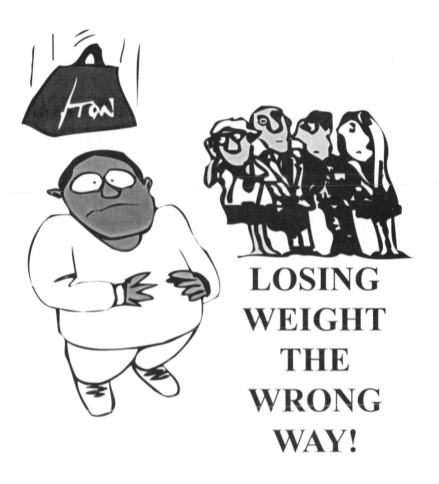

LOSING WEIGHT THE WRONG WAY!

54. *STEP 7*: Trying Exchanges

Practice makes perfect. Repetition helps retention. Calories count. Count calories. Today is the seventh step towards *your control* of diabetes.

When digesting food, the body tries to deny entry of harmful substances (bad things). Ideally we don't eat anything that is bad for us (toxic). Many dietary errors are eliminated at the other end. Occasionally we vomit them up. The kidney can also "void" mistakes.

Persistent errors result in a toxic burden we may or may not notice. Our health bears this burden. Toxic overload produces disease and disease lowers our ability to handle past, present, or future toxic burdens. Too much of anything can eventually become toxic. We all need to eat and do things in moderation. To this degree, all of us are "what we eat."

Diabetics should eat food that is nutritious and avoid, as much as possible, anything that is bad (toxic). The disease "diabetes" limits the body's ability to manage calories (energy). Therefore, your energy level depends on when and how much you eat (in calories). If you eat too many calories, you either gain weight or your blood sugar rises. If you don't eat calories when needed, you run out of gas (hypoglycemia). Counting calories is so important in helping to avoid errors in energy management. High blood glucose and/or high insulin resistance is toxic. To stop further harm, these problems need to remain under control. Tomorrow's health depends on how you take control of your diabetes today.

Unfortunately, you have already accumulated a toxic burden caused by past high blood glucose levels and/or insulin resistance. What damage has already accumulated over time, cannot be entirely eliminated. This makes you, the diabetic, vulnerable to many other diseases and complications. If these other problems are not properly addressed, you only enlarge the toxic burden that can affect your health. It's a vicious cycle. Disease lowers your ability to tolerate dietary errors, and dietary errors (toxic burden) cause disease. It all adds up. Every time you cheat on your diet a piece of **you** (i.e. your body) pays the price.

STEP 7

The sole purpose of a healthy diet is to provide nutrients while minimizing the toxic burden of any dietary mistake. The first step to good health is to stop killing yourself!! It cannot be emphasized enough—pills and shots cannot fix how or what we put in our own mouth (eat). The second step to good health is a good balanced diet (eat right!).

So what is a good diet? The American Diabetic Association dots the "i's" and crosses the "t's" on exactly what is a good diet. Naturally, their diet should be ideal for diabetics. Surprisingly, the total elimination of fat from the diet is not recommended for diabetics. A vegetarian diet can markedly increase blood cholesterol in diabetic patients. The dietary plan for diabetics is spelled out by the "exchange system." To successfully complete this program, you must learn to plan all meals ahead of time. This isn't too hard if you are already doing everything "the same, the same, the same..." This program is easy if you are already recording and counting calories prior to putting anything in your mouth. In other words, you have completed Step 1 through Step 6. So far, nothing you have done was for nothing. Diabetes is not worth dying for. Diet is the first treatment for diabetes.

Goals for STEP 7:

A. You and your doctor have agreed on the following goals:
1) Normal Glucose: Maintaining fasting glucose from 80 to 120 (i.e., 100+20), after meals <140.
2) Calories per Day (six meals per day):_____
3) Target Weight (if losing weight, <3 lbs. per week):_____
4) Daily Exercise (>30 minutes per day):
        What? _____
        Where? _____
        When? _____
        Any Help? _____
5) American Diabetic Assoc. (ADA) exchange diet program (available from most doctors, dieticians, and book stores).

B. Adapting the ADA Exchange System Diet.

#1. Not everything the ADA tells you is true. The ADA is affected by politics. Some of their programs view the word "calories" as politically incorrect. The ADA also suggests that diabetics can eat somewhat like normal people. This is not true. Some dietary items listed in the ADA Exchange System should be deleted. What is there about "no crap" (e.g., juice) that you don't understand?

#2. The ADA suggests "breakfast," "lunch," "dinner," with "snacks" in between. There is no "breakfast," lunch," "dinner" for a diabetic. A good diet has no crappy "snacks." You must eat six small nutritious meals per day. Each meal is adjusted, calorie-wise, for the proceeding activities planned. Every meal is scheduled to balance "energy in" with "energy out." **No big meals** (e.g., dinner).

#3. Your daily calorie count goal determines how many exchanges you can eat in one day. From each exchange list, pick out what you want to eat. Using the correct amount of food from each exchange(s) — take the day's worth of food and pile it on a table (sound familiar?). Divide all this food into 6 small piles and eat these six meals (on time) throughout the day. The same calories per meal should satisfy the same activity levels the same time every day (just different foods are needed). Go to sleep and get up at the same time. The same, the same, the same...

#4. When catastrophe occurs, well-planned activities may have to be canceled. This may include the dietary plans you had for the day. When this happens, skip the planned "exchange" and simply go back to calorie counting. Even on bad days, you still must eat on time. If you can't eat the exchange you had planned, then eat anything that has fiber and the correct calorie count. This prevents hypoglycemia, which is more important than perfectly adhering to the ADA exchange system. Unplanned diet — "bad day" — is the exception rather than the rule.

#5. Write everything down in your food diary. When you see your doctor, discuss any problems you are having. Remember, practice (and planning) makes perfect.

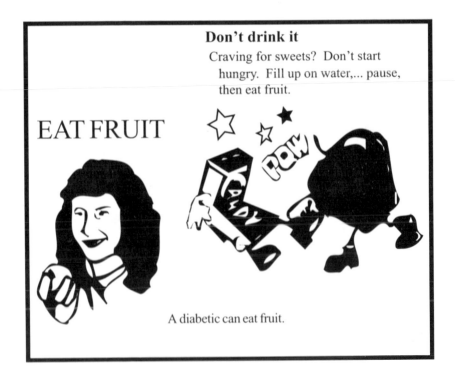

Don't drink it

Craving for sweets? Don't start hungry. Fill up on water,... pause, then eat fruit.

EAT FRUIT

A diabetic can eat fruit.

55. Seeing Drugs in a New Light

Sooner or later, as a diabetic, your doctor will recommend a "pill" for you to take. Your attitude about drugs is important, so read on....

Perceptions about "drugs" are greatly influenced by the mass media. They help form public opinion about drugs. Issues on drugs are easily politicized. Hence, scientific data are easily ignored or exaggerated.

It took many years for science and medicine to overcome the political influence that tobacco had on the "free" press. Dr. Everett Koop (former Surgeon General) was only recently able to correctly classify nicotine as a known addicting substance. Cigarettes were initially marketed to improve health (that was many years ago). It took a long time to correct that mistake.

Unfortunately the process of changing public opinion also generates public confusion. What is a "bad" drug and what is "addiction" are not clear to many people.

So what is a "drug"? A drug is a potent example of a substance that enters our bodies and influences the way we feel (physically or emotionally). Normal food and drink do not have such a rapid, obvious impact on how we usually feel. The difference between food and drugs is not black and white. There are drugs that are less potent and there are foods that seem to have a more obvious impact on how we feel. (There is a continuum between black and white. It's called "shades of gray.")

The difference between "good" drugs and "bad" drugs can also be uncertain (i.e. "gray").

Most prescribed medications, in the right hands, are viewed as "good" drugs. Most illegal drugs are viewed as "bad." Current popular opinion sees most herbal remedies as "good." The government classifies these substances as "food." Some drugs stay controversial. A good example is the current fight to allow marijuana use for medicinal purposes (now legal in California).

In many instances, circumstance dictates what is "good" or "bad."

Step 8

Alcohol is bad for an alcoholic. A glass of wine per day can help prevent some people from having a heart attack. That's good.

A DUI (driving under the influence) is a law that is popularly believed to help address excessive alcohol consumption (i.e. control alcohol abuse). It's popular for politicians to define DUIs with lower and measured alcohol levels. But legally, DUI laws do not confine their interests merely to alcohol levels. These are the laws that address any substance that impairs the functions needed to drive safely. It's the impairment, not the drug, that causes accidents.

A person with a high alcohol level might not be as impaired as a person who mixes marijuana with alcohol. It is well-known that some people can, in fact, develop a high "tolerance" for alcohol. Therefore, alcohol levels are not a very good way to define impairment.

The medical definition of tolerance is met when increasingly large amounts of drugs are needed to produce the same effects (regardless of whether the effects are desirable or undesirable). Concerns for drug abuse occur when patients demand more and more medication to maintain or achieve the drug's effect. But not everyone who develops tolerance is addicted to that drug (or substance). Most people confuse drug tolerance with drug addiction and/or abuse. These words do not mean the same thing.

Drug "withdrawal" refers to symptoms that develop when a drug (or a substance) is no longer being used. Usually, symptoms of withdrawal are well-characterized and, therefore, "withdrawal" is defined by the presence of those symptoms. Ignorance about the symptoms of withdrawal prevents the diagnosis. There are drug withdrawal symptoms that society habitually labels as normal and, therefore, the substance is never recognized as having that problem.

Patients can develop symptoms of withdrawal without ever developing symptoms of tolerance. Drug abusers and drug addictions can exist without problems of withdrawal or tolerance. Obviously, the potential for a drug to be abused is greater when either tolerance and/or withdrawal can easily develop.

Step 8

I define drug abuse as "trouble" with a drug. The definition of "trouble" can be very broad. Obvious examples of trouble are legal ones. Obtaining, using, or distributing illegal drugs and getting caught can cause a lot of "trouble."

Those who advocate that marijuana should be used for medicinal purposes argue that many users' only "troubles" are the legalities of its use. In other words, if marijuana were legal, there wouldn't be any "trouble."

"Trouble," like any other word associated with drug abuse or addiction, can be in the eye of the beholder. Behavioral changes caused by drugs can be considered to be good by one person and not by another. Other "troubles" can include physical ailments associated with continued drug use. "Trouble" can be the time and effort needed to obtain or maintain the drug use. And finally, there is everything in between...

Marijuana is a drug rich in history and politics. Public perception has waxed and waned over many years. Laws passed and enforced are rarely based on the scientific facts known today.

The active ingredient of marijuana is a fat-soluble drug. Because of this, infrequent users have a transient, but measurable, blood level of the drug. Because blood is primarily water, a fat-soluble drug doesn't stay there for long (just like oil stays separate from water).

Only after many months of frequent use does the drug become absorbed into cells that contain fat. Once this has been successfully accomplished, eliminating marijuana from blood levels becomes equally difficult. Even if marijuana usage stops, these cells can now effectively release enough stored drug to maintain blood levels.

Persistent blood levels of marijuana, after all usage has stopped, prevents any possibility of developing withdrawal symptoms. Therefore, it is not possible to know if withdrawal symptoms can even exist with chronic marijuana use. Deciding whether this drug is "good or "bad" based on withdrawal symptoms alone is not practical.

Some early advocates for the legalization of marijuana dropped out because of the development of unusually early and severe emphysema. Remaining advocates blamed government spraying of marijuana plants as the problem. There is plenty of evidence that the way people smoke marijuana is a problem as well. The fact remains that marijuana smoking, like cigarette smoking, can cause wholesale destruction of the lung. The legality of cigarette smoking doesn't make smoking right. The lung problems caused by marijuana smoking would make the legalization troublesome.

Finally, marijuana use can affect how people think. The observation that marijuana use can convert an "A" student into an "F" student is well known. The lack of interest in the real world usually interferes with productivity. The withdrawal into a world influenced by drugs clearly develops in some people under the influence of marijuana smoking. Just because that's what a person now wants doesn't make it right.

Changing the way we feel is not always "bad." Prescribed antidepressants do this, too, and can dramatically improve a person's productivity. However, making people feel better at the expense of productivity can cause a lot of problems.

When is it okay to change how people feel and when isn't it? This can be a complicated issue.

One interesting study showed that musicians, under the influence of marijuana smoking, believed that their music and creativity were enhanced by this drug. However, when the drug use and influence were stopped, and the musicians were allowed to hear taped music that was produced under drug use, their opinions changed. All the musicians preferred the music they produced that had not been influenced by marijuana use. The experiment and their interest in marijuana use both ended.

The decision to use a drug can be influenced by the presence of the drug. When problems from chronic marijuana use develop (e.g., emphysema), many patients fail to stop smoking it. One reason may be that stopping chronic use does not eliminate the drug from the body. Marijuana blood levels remain. The lack of interest in the real world prevents users from being concerned about the consequences of its use. Therefore the decision to stop using the drug may not ever be seriously considered.

STEP 8

It's been my personal experience, as a physician, that getting an alcoholic to stop drinking alcohol is much easier (but still difficult) than getting a marijuana abuser to stop using marijuana. Marijuana tends to rob people of motivation and, therefore, it is very difficult to motivate chronic marijuana users to quit smoking it.

Alcohol, in contrast, is water soluble. Its direct influence on the mind can end when rapid withdrawal occurs. A sober alcoholic can then sometimes be motivated to quit drinking. Additionally, the symptoms of withdrawal caused by rapid withdrawal can help improve motivation to quit..

There are many people who have smoked marijuana without any obvious long-term problems. Many of these people are not unsympathetic to decriminalizing or legalizing marijuana. I have no personal experience with the medicinal value of marijuana. Data on this use is limited. But my overall opinion is that most people do not need to use this drug. It causes more harm than good.

The decision as to whether a drug is "good" or "bad" depends on a variety of things. Diagnosing drug addiction and/or abuse involves the same issues.

To the degree "troubles" develop during the use of drugs, drug addiction or abuse needs to be considered. To the degree patients exert time and energy to obtain drugs, drug addiction or abuse needs to be considered. To the degree that withdrawal symptoms or tolerance can develop with a drug, drug addiction and/or abuse needs to be considered. However, such a definition opens the diagnosis to a wide range of substances. These substances do not simply include "good" or "bad" drugs.

Problems with any substance or abuse can be categorized in many different ways. Problems with drugs can affect the person directly or indirectly. Drugs affect people in different ways. Ultimately, substance abuse is not so much the drug but the impact the drug has. It's either "good" or "bad."

A broader definition of "drugs," drug abuse, and/or drug addiction means that "zero tolerance to drugs" is a stupid solution to a complex problem. Drug abuse and addiction are not black and white problems. Therefore solutions are not that simple, either.

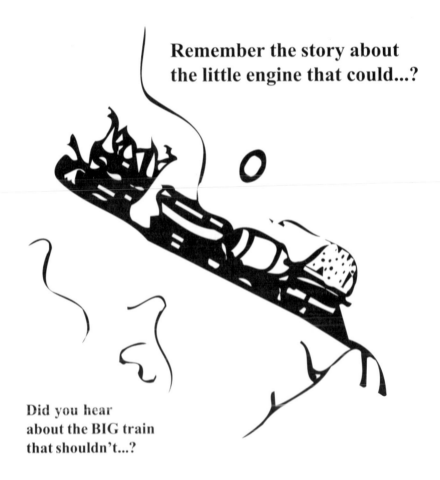

**Remember the story about
the little engine that could...?**

**Did you hear
about the BIG train
that shouldn't...?**

56. The Most Abused Substance in America

Everyone has a desire for something.

Craving for a substance is not always bad or abnormal. Craving for air keeps us breathing. It is an urge that cannot normally be stopped. Thirst is also a craving that eventually becomes very strong when not satisfied. Any strong craving can dominate both thought and behavior. These kinds of cravings are considered normal and tend to help maintain life. An addict has a craving for a substance that is harmful to life rather than one that is needed to sustain life or well-being. Inadvertent exposure to dangerous substances is not the same as deliberate use. Substance abuse is the result of both harmful behavior and harmful substances.

The substance that causes addiction in the highest percentage of users could be considered the "most abused" substance in America. Some substances are notoriously abused by their users. In other words, most if not all, users tend to develop addictive behavior. The drug's influence results in the rapid decline of the user. An infamous example is "crack."

The majority of Americans avoid dangerous and illegal drugs. Hence, the overall impact of illegal drug use is less important than substances that are more commonly used. The "most abused" substance in America is the one that harms the most Americans (because of addiction) rather than the one that has the highest percentage of users who are abusers (e.g., most "crack" users are abusers).

Alcoholism and nicotine addiction are widespread problems. Many more Americans will die from either of these substances than any illegal drugs. Substance abuse is not defined by the legality of the drug but rather the impact the substance has on the user.

In many instances, problems with abuse are determined more by the user than by the substance. Not everyone who drinks becomes an alcoholic. On the other hand, alcoholics tend to abuse any mood altering substance and not just alcohol. It's not uncommon for alcoholics to "quit" drinking by changing to other substances (e.g., illegal drugs) that are then also abused.

Step 8

The suffering caused by substance abuse takes many forms but the underlying problem is always the same. Despite harm from use, abuse (i.e. use) continues (and is actively sought). The tendency to abuse substances is higher if severe withdrawal symptoms have to be endured when substance abuse ends. Nevertheless, the greatest driving force of continued use of abused substances is not the fear of withdrawal but rather the craving to continue to use the substance. Many abused substances have no known withdrawal symptoms.

As a physician, I spend most days trying to keep patients from killing themselves. Everyone has faults that are extremely difficult to eliminate. Some of these problems impact on health. Despite the harmful effects, some "bad habits" cannot easily be controlled.

As mentioned before, nicotine addiction is a common example. Many smokers know they need to quit and want to quit. Some cannot despite all their best intentions. People who fail to quit smoking either have poor will power (e.g., warning) or have a craving for nicotine that is stronger than their "will" to live. The fact that many smokers suddenly quit after their first heart attack reflects that many patients never really put the effort into quitting (i.e. will power). The fact that many smokers die from smoking-related diseases while still smoking reflects how difficult the craving for nicotine can be.

The failure to stop fatal behavior helps identify how dangerous a substance can be.

For me, the most abused substance in America is the substance that has killed more Americans than any other. It is the substance that I spend the most time on every day trying to convince abusers to avoid. Most patients will readily agree to curtail its use when initially confronted with its harmful effects. Few patients return with successful control over its use. Less, maybe; stop, no.

The most abused substance in America has never demonstrated any nutritional or medicinal value. No one was raised to obtain this substance for that reason. Animals never exposed to this substance will not make any attempt to obtain the substance. It is only after exposure to this substance that animals seek this to replace more essential nutrients. More than one half of all Americans demonstrate overwhelming evidence that their use of this substance should end. More than half never stop. Many patients try to control the abuse of this substance by switching to other unhealthy substances (like an alcoholic switching to drugs). The craving for this substance and the addictive behavior for this substance are becoming increasingly more common in this country. This addictive behavior guarantees future sales and some companies will not pass up the opportunity to sell a substance that can guarantee large profits.

Children, in particular, continue to increase their use of this substance. Schools promote its use in exchange for money that is easier to obtain than that from the tax payer. Advertising for this substance exceeds all the money spent on education in this country (including higher eduction). Even athletes are encouraged to obtain this substance. A substance that kills that many people is a powerful drug. Therefore, there is no school that truly has an enforced "no drug zone."

The most abused substance in the fattest country in the world (America), in my opinion, is plain sugar (sucrose).

The sugar substitute, an artificial sweetener most commonly known as NutraSweet, is believed to be 100 times sweeter than sugar. The promise that NutraSweet could safely substitute for the more commonly abused substance sugar has never been proven true. The use of NutraSweet has never demonstrated a decline in the use of sugar. In fact, there is growing evidence that it makes the craving for sweets even worse.

The quantity of sugar consumed has climbed to one-third of a pound of sugar per person per day. In other words, the average American eats one pound of sugar every three days. The average American also eats one pound of NutraSweet in five days.

How many overweight diabetics you know have actually stopped eating sweets completely? Is sugar worth dying for? In America, the answer is yes. And the answer demonstrates how addicted America has become to sugar.

STEP 8

It is a public health disaster that America has failed to recognize its worst vice. Because of this, very little is being done about this problem or to reverse current trends. The mere fact that schools have replaced cigarette machines with even larger numbers of soda machines is predictive that our next generation will do even worse.

It's always the addict who is the last to recognize the problem.

---

10 MINUTES TO CONTROL DIABETES: NO IF'S, AND'S, OR BUT'S!

1. Everyday is the rest of your life.
2. Why you eat affects what you eat.
3. Read one chapter per day, EVERYDAY.
4. Lifelong diet is a lifestyle change.
5. It's not a lifestyle change unless it's done everyday.
6. Spend 10 minutes per day, EVERYDAY, on any new dietary change (e.g., read more, counting calories, finding new things to eat, etc.)
7. Don't spend more than 15 minutes per day on any dietary change. If you spend too much time working on your diet, you can't do it EVERYDAY.
8. Everything does not have to be done in one day.
9. If you don't have 10 minutes EVERYDAY for "paper work," you won't have time to go to the bathroom.
10. You are what you eat if you can't eliminate crap..

---

57. TOO SWEET TO BE TRUE

The failure to stop fatal behavior helps to identify how dangerous addiction can be. Addiction, by definition, is difficult to stop and, therefore, difficult to treat.

Treatment consists of a variety of strategies. But the underlying goal is to make it easier for the addict to avoid the problem substance.

One controversial strategy is a technique used for heroin addicts, using methadone as a substitute narcotic. Heroin addicts are addicted to narcotics.

In order for an addict to be considered a candidate for the methadone treatment, he must be willing to give up the "high" he has sought. They do not merely crave the drug; they normally also enjoy the "high."

A drug problem means that the addict is having trouble because of using the drug. Heroin is an expensive drug and most addicts lose their jobs while "high." This forces the addict to break the law in order to obtain money. To save money, dirty needles that can cause AIDS are reused. The loss of job, children, spouse, and the threat of jail are some of the reasons why heroin addicts reconsider their use of heroin.

The quality of heroin illegally obtained varies tremendously. Heroin addicts can unintentionally overdose and can find themselves injecting substances that will not give them enough narcotic to prevent withdrawal symptoms. A near-death overdose or severe withdrawal symptoms are other reasons a heroin addict may seek help.

The dose of methadone prescribed in a methadone clinic is designed to prevent withdrawal symptoms and reduce the craving for the narcotic to a tolerable level. The methadone dosage is slowly lowered until the user is off all narcotics. Stopping methadone too quickly causes withdrawal symptoms, increased craving for narcotics, and/or both. Therefore, the dosage of methadone is adjusted very slowly.

Heroin addicts want to stop for a reason. Not getting "high" isn't one of them. Methadone does not satisfy the desire to be "high." Patients need to

Step 8

be sufficiently motivated to handle this craving on their own. Most methadone clinic treatments are complemented with counseling (e.g., support groups, etc.).

Methadone clinics allow the prescriber to supervise the use of narcotics. The prescribed medication is free of any contaminants. The threat of AIDS is no longer a problem. The problem of overdose or underdose is also eliminated.

Critics of the methadone treatment cite a variety of reasons why this method of treatment should not be used. Many people find it offensive that tax dollar money is spent giving free narcotics to drug addicts. The alternative for drug addicts is to break into your house and get the money they need. One way or another, the honest folks pay for the drug addicts' habit (including the cost of AIDS). Who said life is fair? It's a lot cleaner and less messy if the drug addict picks this stuff up at the clinic.

Critics are concerned that addicts will not stop using methadone (i.e. narcotics). There are addicts for whom any lowering of the methadone does result in relapse to heroin use. Whether this is because the addict has no intention of stopping or whether the craving is that much harder to control, nobody knows. In any event, most methadone programs do not give narcotics indefinitely. (However, one could argue that we should.)

The treatment of addiction is always difficult. Many heroin addicts fail treatment. There is no pill that can effectively treat the desire for a high without giving a high — which would be no progress towards a normal life.

I feel that the most abused substance in America is sugar. Many people have an uncontrolled craving for sweets. Sugar has a lot of calories and is not filling. Because of this, too many calories are easily consumed and obesity becomes a big problem.

The uncontrolled "sweet tooth" (or sugar addiction) wrecks havoc on the best dietary intentions to lose weight.

NutraSweet was sold to the government and the general public as a safe substitute for sugar. It could satisfy the sweet tooth without the calories, the perfect solution in a country where more than half of its citizens are overweight. Now Americans could have their cake and eat it, too.

The idea of a substitute sweetener for sugar is similar to the idea that methadone is substituting for heroin. Many of the problems of the bad drug (e.g., sugar, heroin), could be fixed by substituting a better drug (e.g., methadone, NutraSweet). This strategy wouldn't necessarily fix the problem, but it would make the problem a lot less severe. In other words, sugar (calories) could be eliminated.

In contrast to a methadone clinic, the use of NutraSweet is not supervised. Patients can therefore easily obtain both NutraSweet and sugar. In fact, manufacturers of desserts and sweets do this all the time.

NutraSweet is a hundred times sweeter than sugar and the net effect is not less sugar, but sweeter sweets. In no way do sweeter sweets curtail the craving of a sweet tooth.

The urgency of trying to reduce the number of calories that the average American eats has allowed the manufacturers of NutraSweet to have their products approved with less rigorous testing for safety. Concerns that this product can cause brain cancer and/or Alzheimer's disease have not been resolved, despite its approval for sale.

There is absolutely no evidence that NutraSweet reduces sugar consumption. In fact, the sugar consumption in America continues to rise. The average American eats a pound of sugar every three days. Now in addition, the average American also eats a pound of NutraSweet in five days.

NutraSweet is not the "methadone" it was thought to be.

One reason for this is that the methadone treatment strategy requires extremely vigorous supervision by the prescriber over the addict. Since heroin is difficult to obtain, methadone becomes a reasonable alternative for some addicts. However, for the sugar addict, NutraSweet simply becomes an added option.

There's a big difference between adding to products rather than substituting one for the other. My patients almost always did better when all sweets and all addictive behavior for sweets was eliminated. The longer abstinence is maintained, the easier it usually gets to maintain. Not everything is

STEP 8

easy. If it were easy, there wouldn't be so many fat people.

Sugar addicts are dying for sweets. If an idea sounds too sweet to be true, it is.

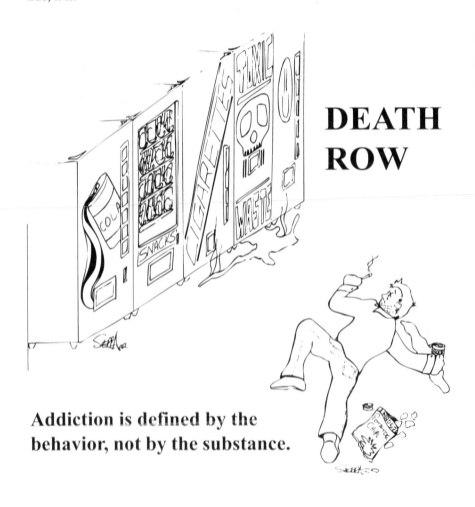

Addiction is defined by the behavior, not by the substance.

58. Licking Sugar Cold-Turkey

Many health problems demand needed changes in behavior. Alcoholics are usually facing a lot of other people's concerns about their drinking. Anyone becomes defensive when they are under attack. The bigger the problem, the more concern people have about that problem. The more concern, the more defensive the alcoholic becomes.

If I ask an alcoholic who is still drinking if he (or she) is able to stop, he might quickly answer, "Yes, I've quit drinking lots of times before."

Over the years as a doctor, I have noticed little clues about human behavior. This short answer suggests a few things. It's subtle, but quitting is not the same as stopping. "Stop" can refer to either "pause" or "quit." Pause means that you stop and then resume. Quitting is stopping forever... and you only do that once. By definition, the answer "I've quit drinking lots of times," is untrue. You can pause (i.e. stop) many times but you can only "quit" once (i.e. bring it to an end).

An alcoholic has an unconscious (but defensive) denial about his lack of control over drinking. The answer "I have quit many times" reflects this. Inherently contradictory, this answer reflects the fact that the addict is usually the last person to realize his/her addiction (or addictive behavior).

Social attitudes play a big role in an alcoholic's behavior. Society does not condone alcoholism. Driving under the influence (DUI) is not legal. Most of society either tolerates or encourages social drinking. (It's also perfectly legal.) Because of this, an alcoholic in denial tries to portray himself as a "social drinker." If a true "social drinker" is asked to stop drinking for medical reasons, he will. Many social drinkers have never been asked to stop before, therefore, some tend to hesitate in responding. Many will question why there is a need to stop (although social drinkers are not particularly confrontational about the subject). If legitimate reasons to stop drinking are presented, the social drinker "quits" (i.e. stops forever) without further counseling.

In contrast, an alcoholic, if asked to stop drinking, quickly becomes defensive. There are two strategies. The first is to volunteer great tales of success on their ability to control drinking (e.g., "I quit drinking many times before"). The other is to become confrontational about the need to stop drinking ("why should I?"). Confrontation about the need to change behavior on a one-to-one basis usually leads to a standstill. Many alcoholics confront the "stop" question with the "I quit many times before" answer. (These tactics allow many alcoholics to continue drinking.) However, if society confronts an alcoholic, continued confrontation doesn't work (especially in front of a judge). Instead, the alcoholic tries to disguise himself as a "social drinker." The conversation goes from "why?" to "can do...," "I can stop drinking," I quit many times before."

Most of us know that what distinguishes a social drinker from an alcoholic is his control over drinking. Though it may be unconsciously, so does an alcoholic. **I hear alcoholics say** *"I quit many times before"* **a lot.** The alcoholic's charade to maintain the disguise of a "social drinker" can become unmanageable. The lies needed to hide the truth can become big enough that even the alcoholic can see past his/her own self deceit (denial) about his or her control over drinking. Recognizing one's own addictive behavior is extremely helpful in ending that behavior.

Alcoholics Anonymous (AA) is the most successful organization in the world to help alcoholics stop drinking. There are twelve steps. The first step for an alcoholic is to stop denying his drinking problem.

Part of AA's success depends on society's attitude not to tolerate alcoholism. Social pressure can be extremely helpful in providing the confrontation needed to force an alcoholic to admit to himself that he is an alcoholic. An alcoholic must confess his addiction.

Another step in AA is that the alcoholic acknowledges that he is powerless to control his drinking. He can't drink "socially" (i.e. in moderation). Therefore, all drinking must stop. No ifs, ands, or buts. **Total** abstinence.

Again, society's attitude about alcoholism helps support this goal of abstinence. It's been well proven that total abstinence is the best treatment for all alcoholics.

STEP 8

In the last five years, I have really been struck by how much a sugar addict (lover of sweets) sounds like an alcoholic (it's also striking how many recovering alcoholics become sugar addicts). This problem usually comes up when patients are either overweight and/or have diabetes.

When confronted with an obvious need to stop using sugar, I usually hear a sugar addict in denial say any one of the following excuses (denials): "I can always lose weight, I've lost weight plenty of times before," "I've quit drinking sodas before and I can do it again," "I can stop using sugar, I've been on plenty of diets before," "I only eat sweets on 'social' occasions," etc., etc.

A sugar addict sounds and behaves just like an alcoholic. Despite the obvious need to avoid sweets, "quitting" reverts back to a brief pause... and his health problems continue to get worse.

The leading cause of death in America is not alcoholism; it's heart attacks. Many of these heart attacks can be traced back to sugar addiction.

A true sugar addict hides his problem just like an alcoholic who tries to look like a "social drinker." Unfortunately, there are few in society who would confront a sugar addict like they would an alcoholic. Most sugar addicts are forced to recognize their problem on their own. Because of this, a lot of addictive behavior for sweets is ignored and left untreated.

Worse yet, in this country, many dieters attempt to control this problem are actually discouraged. Try staying on a healthy diet yourself. America does not support sugar abstinence.

For every known alcoholic I see in the office, I probably see ten people who cannot control their consumption of sweets. **I hear** *"I quit many times before"* **a lot.** Like an alcoholic, sugar addicts can be fairly easy to recognize.

Despite the attitudes of society, a small number of sugar addicts recognize their addictive behavior. Once this important first step is achieved, abstinence becomes the goal.

Though going "cold turkey" can be tough, licking the sugar addiction is still worth the effort. Most successful dieters feel, look, and do better. Sugar, like alcohol, is not worth dying for.

It's a shame that society doesn't do more to help with this problem.

TRYING ...

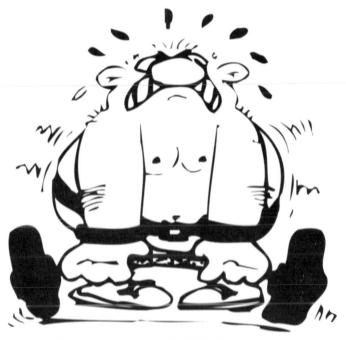

DOES NOT COUNT.

59. Killing the Ones We Love

Mankind has found incredibly clever and efficient ways to kill people. The mark the terrorists left in New York City pales compared to what we are doing to our children.

Children mimic adult behavior. Your habits become their habits. "Do as I say, not as I do" never works. When I was a kid, a soda was a rare treat. My parents never drank sodas. Milk and water were the only choices at school.

When my generation became adults, they all drank more sodas than before. Our kids are drinking sodas, too. They are drinking at least as much, if not more, than their parents do. And children are much smaller than we are.

Well, some of them are.

The percentage of obese children is at a record high. This percentage of overweight children has been doubling since the 1970s. Only now, doubling takes half the time (ten years). We know that fat kids will become fat adults. The number of overweight adults can only go up. The average age of onset for obesity can only go down.

Diabetes is the second most expensive diagnosis in America. Obesity and diet are the greatest predictors of disease. This is why the combination of diabetes and obesity is referred to as "*diabesity*." The growth of "diabesity" has increased so much that it will become the most expensive epidemic America has ever faced. Studies clearly show, in the last ten years, that all age groups have doubled the rate of obesity. Very large studies have shown that a twenty pound weight gain will increase the chances of developing diabetes by at least twenty fold. It is no longer uncommon for young children to be as overweight as their parents, only these children are many years younger.

Another important factor for diet is twentieth-century technology. Mass marketing and propaganda can rapidly change the behavior of entire

Step 8

societies. If the Nazis in Germany, with propaganda, could turn an entire civilized nation into a killing machine, why can't soda companies double their sales in less than twenty years? The answer is that they did. The average American eats (consumes) a pound of sugar every three days and a third of this comes from sodas. It doesn't take a rocket scientist to figure out that soda consumption is contributing to the epidemic of "diabesity."

Many years ago, the American Lung Association realized that 90% of lung disease and lung cancer was related to cigarette smoking. This being their main concern, they decided to spend billions of dollars on the same venues that tobacco companies were using to increase sales, which is advertising. If tobacco companies can persuade more people to smoke, why couldn't the Lung Association persuade people to quit? The answer is they can. While cigarette sales around the world are flourishing (and growing), sales in America have not. The number of smokers who have quit has risen to record numbers.

The Lung Association could have, like the American Diabetic Association (ADA), spent the money it raised on research to treat disease. However, the Lung Association realized how much simpler it would be to prevent disease. The majority of lung patients suffered from self-inflicted disease that could be stopped with good advertising.

In contrast, the ADA has done little to prevent Americans from overeating. Most of their money goes towards lobbying for money and research to treat disease. Diet neglected, "diabesity" continues to rise.

Thanks to the American Lung Association, lung cancer is no longer the leading cancer death in men. While there has been some improvement in lung cancer treatment, these improvements are not significant. Therefore, the prevention of lung disease by effective marketing has been the main reason cancer deaths are falling.

An ounce of prevention is still worth a pound of cure.

Good marketing is effective advertising. Good marketing changes people's behavior.

Soda companies spend more on marketing than America does on all education combined (including college tuition). Soda sales continue to rise. Every indication suggests that our children will do even worse than their predecessors.

While some of us still tell our children to eat their vegetables, more times than not, they are eating fast food instead. They are also drinking more sodas than ever before.

Cigarette machines have been replaced by soda machines at public schools.

Our kids are becoming fatter, faster than ever before, and eating habits continue to worsen. It's not only marketing that is doing this; it's also the way that parents eat and drink.

The most dangerous threats facing America are not terrorists. The greatest threat is the way we eat and the way we teach our children to eat. If you do not want to improve your diet or health for your own sake, could you not consider doing so for your children's or grandchildren's sakes? Children will never eat better if adults won't.

Thousands of Americans died in the World Trade Center attack. Millions will die from "diabesity." Eat like an American; die like an American; that's what "diabesity" is.

More grown children than ever before are having heart attacks, strokes, and bypass surgery before their elderly parents do. This same generation will also have to care for an aging population that is disproportionately large compared to previous generations.

A good diet is not just what **you** eat; it's what your whole family eats.

If America is to remain strong and secure, there must be people well enough to carry on the American dream. The real threat to America is from within. We are killing the ones we love with bad diet. Each generation continues to do far worse than the one before.

60. Dieters Can't Diet Alone, *Especially at Home*

It always amazes me how dieters can tell all of their relatives and friends that they are "on a diet," yet everyone will still offer them food and drink that they should be avoiding. I think it can be very discouraging to be on a diet when no one who cares about you actually helps you stay on that "diet."

In contrast, if an alcoholic announced he or she wants to stop drinking, few would offer another drink. In fact, many concerned loved ones would avoid drinking in front of the alcoholic in recovery. Yet if the alcoholic announced he or she needed to lose weight, most would offer that alcoholic some dessert. It seems peculiar that society doesn't want people to drink themselves to death but continually encourages them to eat themselves to death. The means (how you die) have no effect on the end (you are still dead). Any fatal mistake will be that person's last one.

Addiction is not caused by the substance. Addiction is defined by the behavior of the addict. When a person has a craving for any harmful substance and yet still uses that substance (despite the harm it causes), that person is demonstrating addictive behavior. A diabetic who eats or drinks any substance that harms blood glucose control and continues to do so despite the harm it causes demonstrates addictive behavior.

Most alcoholics and drug addicts can expect society's encouragement to avoid the substances they crave. Dieters are much less likely to get this same support. Home-cooked meals, holidays and any social function rarely offer foods and drinks that a dieter can enjoy. Yet commonly, an alcoholic can attend these same functions without being confronted with alcohol. Restaurants are particularly good in keeping the bar separate from the dinner table and yet offer few choices for the dieter.

But a craving for food or drink that the dieter has, which needs to be avoided, can be as strong as the craving that an alcoholic has for alcohol. Few dieters who have been overweight for many years can succeed without getting help from somebody. For people who are married, the spouse can be the most important determining factor. The idea of marriage is to love, honor and cherish with the untimely death ("death do us part") of one spouse being the only obstacle. Any spouses who refuse to help a dieter who desperately needs to lose weight or control disease cannot possibly have much concern for the person to whom they are married. I believe that this is a spouse who needs a divorce. "Death do us part" does not mean that you help set an earlier date. Dieters can't diet alone, especially at home.

Grown children who live in the home of a dieter and taunt his/her efforts to improve his/her diet need an eviction notice. Young children who complain about improved and healthier meals will learn that they cannot starve themselves to death even if they tried. There is nothing wrong with children eating healthy foods.

As you can see, I am adamant that a dieter should never diet alone. Those closest to the dieter have a moral obligation to care for those they love. Helping people eat to live, rather than living to eat, is an obligation, not an act of charity. In the home of an alcoholic, everyone concerned understands that alcohol would not be stored or consumed in the home. The same support should be offered to dieters. This means that spouses and children need to be on the same "diet." Junk food and sodas should not be brought into the home of someone on a "no crap" diet.

Dieters can't diet alone, especially at home.

A diet for life can sustain the entire household and not just the dieter. It makes no sense for a dieter to live in a home where others have no concern for his or her well-being. That sounds pretty tough. But actions speak louder than words. People who care about others should show it and not just talk about it. If one member of the family is to succeed, the rest of the family needs to support him/her and act like it (by eating like it), especially at home.

In most homes where dietary changes are absolutely necessary, such as those required by a diabetic, there will definitely be others in the home who need to be on the same diet. They just don't know it yet.

Diabetes type 2 runs in families. This is an eating disorder that runs in families rather than simply a genetic disorder. A diabetic Type 2 who im-

STEP 8

poses his/her proper diet on his/her children is greatly reducing the chances that any of these children will also develop diabetes Type 2.

Sometimes it is the child who needs to be on the diet and not the parents. Diabetes type 1 tends to strike children and this type does not run in families. Therefore, his/her parents will never develop diabetes Type 1. Nevertheless, if parents truly want their child to do well with his/her diet, parents need to be, as strictly, on the same diet, as well. "Do as I say rather than what I do" never works, especially with children.

Dieters can't diet alone, especially at home. More than half of all Americans need to change the way they eat. Less than half do. It is the majority that kills all efforts of the minority to succeed. And it is simply not right, especially at home.

HOME SWEET HOME

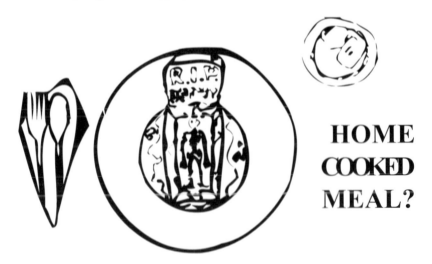

HOME
COOKED
MEAL?

61. Goals for *STEP 8* (Where Do We Go From Here?)

Life is always a battle. That's no reason to quit fighting. Most of us grow old, get sick, get wiser, and die. Some are not that fortunate. They die young and without experience. Today is the eighth step towards *your control* of diabetes.

    The battle of diet is to not lose ground. The war ends when you die. It took your whole life to become a diabetic. It will take the rest of your life to control your diabetes. If it hadn't been for diabetes, you probably wouldn't be working so hard to take care of yourself. If you would stop and think for a moment — i t's really something you should have been doing in the first place (eat right, exercise, and control weight). But before, you never bothered. Now you do!! In this way, diabetes is somewhat of a blessing in disguise. It's only human to take good health for granted. And it's only wise, not to.

    Now you face the endless struggle of staying on your diet. Don't give up on your health and life. Don't quit, don't quit, don't quit...(have we mentioned "no crap?" — what is there about "NO" that you don't understand?, the "N" or the "O" ??).

Goals for STEP 8 (where do we go from here?):

Review: *49. Feet Physics and Good Footwear; 46. Keeping Diabetic Feet; 48. Polyneuropathy: Battle Lines Drawn for Feet; 51. Preventing More than Heart Attacks;* and *53. Living Longer, Hearing Less.*

A. Never stop looking for improvement in diet. Diabetes gets worse. Therefore, diet must keep getting better. This won't make you younger, but it will help you maintain glucose control and live longer. It's important to remember what your goals are. If you establish goals that cannot be met, you are doomed to fail. (Staying young and living forever are good examples.) But whatever goals you are trying to achieve, knowledge is your greatest asset. This means reading, thinking, consulting, and learning. What resources can you find?

1. On the American Diabetic Association (ADA) Exchange Diet: Review Step 7. Go to the library/bookstore for cookbooks/exchange lists. Look for reputable sources. Stay away from best-seller diet books that won't help keep you alive and healthy — (no one denies you can lose weight on a bad diet). Anything (this includes "reputable" sources) that contradicts what your doctor has recommended, discuss it with him/her before changing your diet. Just because the ADA, AHA, etc. have "experts," doesn't mean it is right for you.

2. On Weight Control, review these chapters: *14. The Battle of the Bulge; 60. Dieters Can't Diet Alone, Especially at Home; 59. Killing the Ones We Love;* and *13. Fats, Fads, Facts, & Fiction.* Contact TOPS (1-800-932-8677) or Weight Watchers (1-800-651-6000). Review *22. Carefully Counting with a Calorie Counter; 17. Simply Read a Food Label;* and *21. The Means and the Goal.*

3. On Exercise, review: *36. Dying to Run.* Try joining an exercise club or class. Consider home equipment or nearby partner. If possible, DON'T DO IT ALONE.

4. On Diabetic Foot Care, review chapters on feet care: *49. Feet Physics and Good Footwear; 46. Keeping Diabetic Feet;* and *48. Polyneuropathy: Battle Lines Drawn for Feet.* MAKE SURE YOU CONTACT YOUR PHYSI-CIAN FOR ANY CUT, CALLUS, OR FOOT PAIN (no look, no see).

5. On Good Cholesterol, review: *43. The Gospel on Cholesterol; 39. Fixing Links You Can Fix;* and *42. Suddenly It's a Heart Attack.* If you are pre-scribed medication, make sure you take it for the rest of your life. There is no such thing as temporary lipid-reducing medication (there is no such thing as

temporary diabetes). Read *51. Preventing More Than Heart Attacks.*

6. On Preventing Hypoglycemia, review: *3. When You Run Out of Gas, You Run Out of Go.* Your physician should be consulted if this problem persists. Medication changes may be needed if you are not missing meal times or needed calories. To avoid skipping meals, have backup plans for food emergencies: Review *26. Y'all void' Missing a Meal Now, Yuh Hear?.* Qualified dietitians can help find new ideas. Talk to other diabetics and then your doctor. Review *30. Dieters on the Run.*

7. On "The same, the same, the same...," review Step 6.

8. On the sweet tooth and other big vices, review: *55. Seeing Drugs in a New Light; 56. The Most Abused Substance in America; 57. Too Sweet to Be True;* and *58. Licking Sugar, Cold-Turkey.*

9. On Counting Calories, review Step 3: *22. Carefully Counting with a Calorie Counter; 21. The Means and the Goal;* and *17. Simply Read a Food Label.*

10. On Quality of Food: Eat a little of a lot rather than a lot of a little. There are some great tips on finding better food in *22. Carefully Counting with a Calorie Counter.* This chapter is reeeeeal important. Review Step 2; *34. The Do's and Don'ts of Eating; 18. Nearer the Needle, Further the Forest; 23. The Laws of Physics Apply to You Too;* and *17. Simply Read a Food Label.*

B. If you're smoking, it's time to start working on quitting. As with diabetes, you don't always have to change overnight (cold-turkey). Talk to your doctor about small steps you can take towards quitting (e.g., make your house "NO" smoking — i.e. smoke outside). Review *41. Dead People Don't Smoke.*

Questions commonly asked by patients:

Why can't I lose any more weight? First be sure you should still be trying. Discuss this with your physician. Do not set unrealistic or unsafe goals. Assuming you should still be trying to lose weight, there are two important points you need to remember: First, sooner or later, if you are on a low enough calorie count, you will lose weight (do not starve — it will kill you). Secondly, increase exercise **and activity** to burn more calories. This will help lose weight. Do not underestimate the sedentary lifestyle that you have become accustomed to. Examples include: electric windows in your car (we don't even "roll" down our windows anymore — we push a button); driving 10 minutes looking for a parking space close to the store (to avoid walking?); not only watching too much TV, we won't even get up to change the channel (we'll only get up to search for the remote); etc., etc...

Think real hard how to increase your activity level from where it is now (not just increasing exercise). When's the last time you took the stairs instead of the elevator or escalator? As my mom would say: stop watching TV, go play outside.

Questions I might ask you:

Do you have any symptoms of heart problems?
Have you had any symptoms of hypoglycemia?
How do you treat and prevent hypoglycemia?
How do you handle unplanned events that interfere with planned meals?
Are you having any problems with glucose, diet, weight, or exercise?
Do you know all your medication bottles?
Are you finding new things to eat?
Are you eating six times a day?

62. Drug Experiments and Experience

In order to sell a drug as a drug, the FDA (Food and Drug Administration) requires that a drug be proven safe and effective. Effective for what? Initially, effective for its intended design (indication). Once a drug is proven safe, there is no harm using the same drug for other purposes.

Drugs can be classified by their intended use (as approved by the FDA). For example, drugs used to treat epilepsy are viewed as "seizure" drugs (actually, anti-seizure). However, many of these drugs become popular for reasons not related to their original indication.

Neurotonin is a seizure drug. The most popular reason the drug is being used is for pain control (not seizure control). Pain caused by a pinched or irritated nerve (i.e. the wires from the nerves to the body) can be better treated with this drug rather than with pain control drugs. Except for cost, side effects from Neurotonin are extremely rare.

Mysoline is another seizure drug. Its most popular use is to treat tremor (fine shaking movements). Before using this drug, blood pressure medicine was used to treat tremor. Both drugs can be helpful in some cases.

Valproic acid, an old seizure drug, can be used to treat manic depression. The first and best drug prior to this was Lithium. However, Lithium can harm kidney function and patients with poor kidney function cannot use Lithium. Valproic acid is a very effective alternative.

Several seizure drugs (antidepressants and blood pressure medications, as well) can prevent migraines. However, what works for one patient might not work for another. These medications must be tried for several months to determine if an effective response has occurred.

Obviously, many other drugs have found "new" purpose as well. Some of these drugs are very old and only recently have found new uses.

Quinine was used to treat and prevent malaria. Quinine, with or without theophylline (an asthma drug), is used to treat leg cramps that can occur when trying to sleep.

New drugs can rapidly find new purposes. There is a large class of blood pressure medications called ACE inhibitors. These drugs are widely used to treat high blood pressure (their intended use). However, their role has become much more important in treating congestive heart failure and preventing kidney failure. They also reduce the risk of a heart attack more than expected (based on improvement in blood pressure). This discovery had led to a whole new line of research to prevent heart attacks.

The world's number one selling class of drugs is arthritis medicine. Arthritis medicine can also treat pleurisy (inflammation of the lining around the lung/heart). Gout and migraines can be quickly cooled down in some patients with high doses of these drugs.

Alternative uses for drugs can be so widespread that the original intention for the drug is completely forgotten. FDA approved valium as a muscle relaxer for back pain. The majority of prescriptions filled are for anxiety (nervousness). Antidepressants (drugs indicated for depression) can also be used to treat anxiety. These drugs are used for insomnia as well. Valium can also stop a seizure in an emergency.

Alternative uses for medication can sometimes be used in combination with indicated drugs to boost the indicated drugs' effectiveness. Tagamet, a stomach medication, can help treat hives (allergic reaction). Tagamet boosts the effectiveness of an antihistamine. However, the primary drug for allergic reaction is still an antihistamine.

No effect, no side affect. Side affects are common. Side affects (unintended consequences) can be good (huh?). They can also be bad. This depends on the patient and problem. Aspirin, as a blood thinner, can cause bleeding and prevent heart attacks. Aspirin is bad for a patient with a stomach ulcer. Aspirin is good for someone having a heart attack.

Before FDA approval, new drugs are tried on people enrolled in experimental protocol. Experience with new drugs in people is limited to a small number (thousands). Once a drug is approved for its intended use and successfully marketed, the number of people on that medication goes to millions. New side affects are discovered with time. Rarely can a drug with FDA approval be absolutely safe. Aspirin does kill people. Data are published on any problems associated with any drug. Problems associated with medication must be weighed against its intended purpose.

But there are no guarantees that a drug will help you or harm you.

Testimonials about unexpected improvement for other ailments are reported and published worldwide. Many of these testimonials are never proven any better than herbal remedies. Nevertheless, weighing in their favor is FDA approval for marketing purposes. Any FDA-approved drug has been heavily tested for safety and purity before being released. Popular testimonials usually led to further research and testing. Some are proven false and some true. New indications for old drugs require FDA testing before formal FDA approval for such new purpose.

FDA approval is very expensive. Therefore, many medications proven to be effective for alternative uses never officially receive FDA approval for those uses. Once a drug is approved for sale by the FDA, it can be prescribed for any use. Many manufacturers find it cheaper to sell the drug for other uses without FDA approval.

Knowledge about medication is never complete. Therefore, FDA approval is not all-encompassing. Safety records are established only to the degree possible. To complicate things further, medications are routinely mixed together. The effect of combining different drugs is even less known and the problems associated with combination therapy are obviously more complicated.

Medical knowledge is never complete.

Medicine and math are both scientifically-based fields. Math is an exact science; medicine is not. With enough data, one can precisely (statistically) predict the odds of any effect or side effect. But no one can know the effect a drug has on an **individual** until that person takes the drug.

Drug experience and experiments never end.

As more and more drugs are being made and as uses for drugs continue to expand, more and more people will be taking medication. FDA approved uses should not be taken as the only reason to be on that drug. FDA approval is never a guarantee of safety. In medicine, there are no guarantees.

Step 9

Good drugs are medications that do more good than harm. Any drug that causes more harm than good is bad. The trick is finding the right one for you. Sooner or later, you will need medication to ease suffering or prolong life. Life without medication, for most people, would be worse.

Trial and error can bring reward. Risk is part of everyday life. There is a risk in starting your car. The risk is low enough to drive to where you want to go. If you knew for sure that on that day you would have an accident, you wouldn't drive. But you cannot predict the future. Never driving forward is a poor route for a risk-free life.

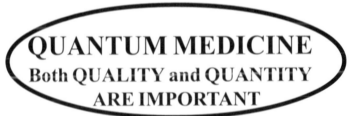

QUANTUM MEDICINE
Both QUALITY and QUANTITY
ARE IMPORTANT

Hard pill to swallow?

Step 9

63. It May Not Be What You Think

Presumably you take medications to help preserve your health. The fact is that medications may serve different people in different ways. Both *effects* and *side effects* of drugs can vary from person to person. A drug for one may not be acceptable for another. Medical care has to be individualized to each person's needs.

Side effects of medication are, by definition, considered to be undesirable. You take a medication for its effects; the side effects come along for the ride.

However, side effects of medications can become advantageous in some circumstances. "One man's trash is another man's treasure." In these cases, the side effect becomes the effect and the effect becomes the side effect. (Got that?)

A generation has forgotten that aspirin was an important drug used to lower temperatures (i.e. treat fevers). "Take two aspirins and call me (the doctor) in the morning" was an old adage that referred to aspirin's frequent use. The discovery that aspirin can sometimes cause Reye's Syndrome has caused physicians to recommend Tylenol for fever. It is no longer recommended that young people use aspirin to treat fever.

For years, aspirin was the **mainstay** for arthritis. Today, again, aspirin has fallen onto hard times. NSAIDs (nonsteroidal antiinflammatory drugs) have almost completely replaced aspirin in treating arthritis. These drugs are more effective, have fewer side effects, and can be taken less often. Examples of these drugs include Advil and Aleve.

One side effect of aspirin is that it can decrease the ability of blood to clot. For years, this problem was considered anything from an unnoticed nuisance to a life-threatening bleeding problem. Surgeons prefer elective surgery so they can advise patients to stop taking aspirin several days before the operation. Increased bleeding is a noticeable problem during surgery in patients who have recently taken aspirin.

However, it has been discovered that aspirin can dramatically reduce the chances of having a heart attack. Researchers were able to show that a blood clot in the artery of the heart was the main cause of heart attacks. Furthermore, studies on aspirin showed dramatic reduction in blood clotting factors that, in turn, caused heart attacks.

Another factor discovered about heart attacks is that the undesirable clot tends to occur in areas of the blood vessel where there is inflammation. Therefore, aspirin can reduce heart attacks in two ways: it can reduce inflammation *and* prevent clot formation.

According to a manufacturer's label (e.g., Bayer), the uses for aspirin are "fast, safe, temporary relief of headache pain, muscular aches and pain, aches and fever... and minor aches and pain of arthritis." No mention of the prevention of heart attacks.

Today, aspirin use is on the rise again. Its current use differs markedly from days past. It is used to provide significant protection against heart attacks. It is strongly recommended for many patients who are at risk for heart disease. A generation ago, no one would have ever dreamed that aspirin would be used for what we are using it for today. One of its "old" side effects has now become one of its most important therapeutic effects.

Medications and their side effects are important research tools. Understanding why aspirin is so helpful against heart attacks helps us understand how heart attacks occur. Many medications with widespread use are later found to have better uses than originally planned.

All medications in this country require FDA (Federal Drug Administration) approval. This process requires that the manufacturer tells the government what the drug is for and what its side effects are. Once a drug is released, this becomes common knowledge.

However, the reason a doctor writes a prescription may not have anything to do with what the drug is approved for by the FDA. Sometimes side effects of medication become their greatest assets.

Blood pressure medications are by prescription only. These medications have been shown to reduce the risk of heart attacks in hypertensive (high blood pressure) patients. This decreased risk of heart attacks with most medications corresponds with the reduction of blood pressure. Therefore, one can calculate an expected reduction of heart attacks with any new blood pressure medication that is introduced.

Unexpectedly, a whole class of blood pressure medications has the side effect of lowering the risk for heart attacks beyond expected results (based on blood pressure control). This class is known as ACE inhibitors. The question is asked "how and why."

These drugs were designed to inhibit enzymes found in the kidney that were believed to cause high blood pressure. Side effects, good in this case, from these medications have led researchers to discover that these same enzymes are in the arteries that feed the heart. We are now beginning to learn how the inflammation (that aspirin helps to block) starts in arteries.

Another side effect of ACE inhibitors is its effects on the kidneys. Researchers have been able to show that hypertension damages kidneys even if blood pressure is now under good control with medications. High blood pressure — with or without treatment — is a common cause of kidney failure and dialysis. So is diabetes.

ACE inhibitors can directly protect kidneys from damage associated with hypertension and/or diabetes. Since ACE inhibitors are fairly unique in this regard, their role in protecting kidney function will probably supercede their ability to lower blood pressure.

Finally, many patients who have had or now have congestive heart failure have been shown to live substantially longer when placed on ACE inhibitors.

Common knowledge is that ACE inhibitors are "blood pressure" medications. Many patients (e.g., diabetics) mistakenly believe that being on these medications is solely for that purpose. Many patients stop their medication, check their blood pressure, and mistakenly conclude that they no longer need this medication.

Naturally, if patients are on these medications for reasons other than hypertension, checking blood pressure serves no useful purpose in deciding whether the medication should be continued.

Step 9

Why someone else is on a drug may not have anything to do with why you are on the same drug. Drug indications (FDA approval) may also not apply to you. If you do not think you should be on a medication, the first question you need to ask is "Why am I on this drug?"

When you seek medical care, you seek advice and knowledge. Most importantly, you seek care for your particular situation. Starting medications is a decision made by both doctor and patient. Stopping medication should be done in the same manner.

If you want to stop a medication, you need to see your doctor. You need to determine **all** the reasons you were taking that particular medication. It may not be what you think.

QUANTUM MEDICINE
MEIJER'S UNCERTAINTY PRINCIPLE
Good medical advice can either be vaguely right
or precisely wrong.
It cannot be both.

Hard pill to swallow?

64. Easy Overdose

Advertisers and manufacturers want you to believe that one product is better than another, even if the two products are essentially the same. There are many medications that actually contain the exact same active ingredients. When people are dissatisfied with a medication, other medications are tried in its place. Without care, this can become dangerous.

For example, acetaminophen is the active pain reliever and temperature-lowering ingredient in the brand Tylenol. Most people do not realize that an overdose of acetaminophen can rapidly destroy the liver. Liver failure results in death. An already damaged liver (e.g., from hepatitis or alcohol) can be destroyed with an even lower dose than the usual lethal dose of acetaminophen. Children and elderly patients are more vulnerable to an overdose of acetaminophen. If acetaminophen doesn't work at the recommended dose, it is not wise to simply take more. Remember—more is not necessarily better.

The following is a partial list of products that are available without prescription. **All** these products contain acetaminophen: Aspirin-free Excedrin and Extra-Strength Excedrin (caplets and geltabs), Aspirin-free Anacin, Gelpirin Tablets, Goody's Extra Strength Headache Powder, Goody's Extra Strength Pain Relief Tablets, all Tylenol products, Vanquish Caplets, Actifed Cold & Sinus medications, Allerest No Drowsiness Tablets, Benedryl Allergy, Maximum Strength Comtrex Allergy-Sinus medications, Dimetapp Allergy Sinus Caplets, Drixoral Allergy Sinus Extended Release Caplets, Sinarest, Sine-Aid, Sine-Off, Sinutab, Sudafed, Children's Panadol Chewable Tablets, Genapap Infant Drops, Infants Feverall, Tempra Tablets and Syrup, Actifed Cold & Sinus, Alka-Selzer Plus, Contact, Coricedin, Robitussin, TheraFlu, Triaminic, Vicks Nyquil, Midol, and Unison with pain-relief Nighttime Sleep Aid.

The following prescription medications also **all** contain acetaminophen: Co-Gesic, Darvocet, Esgic, Fioricet, Hydrocet, Lorcet, Lortab, Percocet, Propacet, Roxicet, Sedapap, Tylox, Vicodin, and Wygesic. Please remember, these are only *partial* lists.

Parents or patients switching from one of these products to another without waiting for the first product to wear off can cause increasingly higher doses of acetaminophen delivered to the liver. Unfortunately, this happens more often than you might think. Do not mix drugs (over the counter or prescribed) without consulting your physician or pharmacist. Did you know that if a child were to eat an entire bottle of Flintstone vitamins at one time that the child would die without emergency treatment? Do not assume that excessive amounts of any product are harmless. Check with poison control (911 can help find the number). Very little is known about the consequences of many excessive herbal and "natural" concoctions or their interactions with prescribed medication. The fatal results of Flintstone vitamins should serve as a warning to be cautious with all medications, even vitamins and minerals.

A prescription drug called Seldane was used for many years. Rare deaths were finally associated with Seldane use. Eventually, it was discovered that there were a few other medications that, when taken, could cause levels of Seldane in the bloodstream to suddenly rise and become toxic in the unfortunate few. Further research discovered that grapefruit juice could cause the same problem. Researchers were able to modify Seldane into a new product called Allegra. Seldane has since been taken off the market. Allegra, new and improved Seldane, does not have this problem.

An overdose of any medication can occur in ways you cannot imagine. All medications need to be used carefully. If an accidental or intentional overdose is discovered, call poison control. Poison control will need the age, height, weight, dosage of all drugs taken, and the time of ingestion when you call. This includes prescribed and over the counter medications. Medical history of illnesses (e.g., hepatitis, etc.) or conditions (e.g., alcoholism, etc.) need to be provided (if known). Even food and drinks (e.g., grapefruit) may become an issue to factor in.

A medication error can be deadly. Before you combine any medications, or increase the dosage, check with your doctor of pharmacist.

It can be a lot easier to overdose than you think.

Post near the telephone:
Poison Control _____.

ALL NATURAL BEVCO. SODAS

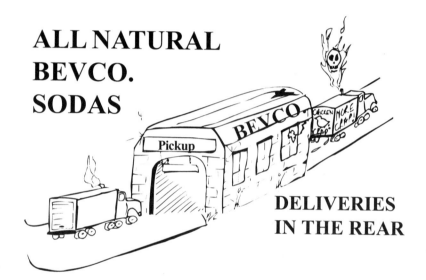

DELIVERIES IN THE REAR

Cola is water with brown crap in it.

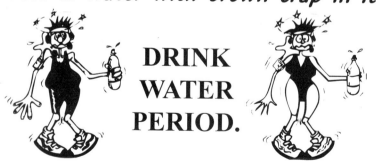

DRINK WATER PERIOD.

Step 9

65. Distinguishing Depressed from Depression

Everyone has feelings. Hunger, anger, worry (anxiety), sadness, and happiness are all feelings we can have. Is it normal for you to control feelings? Most people will answer "yes" but the correct answer is "no." You can decide what you believe in (e.g., try to view the cup as half full) but not how you feel (e.g., on a bad day, the cup feels half empty). Most people confuse beliefs with feelings.

If a crazy man held you hostage with a gun and told you to sit down and shut up, what would you do? If you believe he would harm you, you would sit down and shut up. If he also demanded that you be happy and relaxed, you could not. You could smile but you cannot actually *feel* happy under those circumstances. This is a good example of this important point. We control our behavior and beliefs (attitude) but not our feelings.

The medical word "depression" is a disorder where a person's feelings have changed and are no longer normal (for them). The illness "depression" has two other basic components — severe fatigue and sleep disturbances (insomnia). Examples of changes in feelings (out of character) include: excessive worrying (anxiety about things that are not normally worried about); increased irritability (new temper); urge to cry for no apparent reason (or uncontrollably crying); loss of interest in social or pleasurable activities (e.g., sex); decreased concentration; change in appetite (hunger is a feeling); a new desire to want to run away from problems or stress (i.e. intolerance for daily tasks); less initiative to do things (i.e. don't feel like doing anything); and/or a new desire to be left alone under a rock (i.e. unnatural solitude).

The concept that feelings are preset is not something most people consider. Imagine two different people who undergo the same sad and stressful event: for example, their homes burn down. One is naturally tearful (i.e. homesick) and the other is naturally stoic (i.e. it's just a house that can be rebuilt). These two individuals naturally have different feelings. What would be abnormal is if the stoic person were now to become easily "homesick."

Step 9

The fact is that stress is in the eye of the beholder. Stress is greatly influenced by beliefs (e.g., value of the house) and by feelings we normally have. Increased stress can be caused by abnormal feelings rather than by increasingly worse circumstances.

Normally when we have severe fatigue, we have no trouble sleeping. Depression is one of the few disorders where someone is exhausted but still cannot sleep well (usually wakes up and can't go back to sleep). Usually illnesses that cause fatigue will commonly also cause one to sleep excessively. Fatigue with insomnia is depression until proven otherwise.

An analogy to depression is diabetes. Just as we don't control our feelings, we don't control our blood glucose. Our bodies control this for us. Diabetics have a chemical imbalance of blood glucose. Outside factors, such as diet,, can influence the blood glucose of diabetics. However, the underlying problem is that blood glucose control is not normal. Many patients mistakenly believe that diet causes diabetes. It does not. Diet can help control blood glucose but it does not determine whether or not you have diabetes.

Mood and feelings can also be influenced by outside events (funeral, pay raise, etc.). Normal feelings of sadness (i.e. "depressed") should not be confused with the medical word "depression." Mood can also be influenced by body chemistry (e.g., illnesses). The vulnerability to develop the illness "depression" increases during stressful events. True clinical depression is not caused by such events. The normal sadness of a funeral ("I feel depressed") does not cause the illness depression. It simply makes the illness depression more noticeable.

As with diabetes, the illness depression is caused by a chemical imbalance within our body. This illness is located in the area of the brain that controls mood or feelings. As with diabetes, medication is needed to reestablish normal body chemistry.

Since we cannot control feelings, we cannot cause depression. Most depressed patients try to control these new inappropriate feelings, not realizing that they cannot succeed. This results in most depressed patients not seeking medical care even though they do not feel well. Besides fatigue and

Step 9

insomnia, a variety of other painful symptoms can also be caused by depression. Contrary to popular belief, pain is always "in your head."

If you break your leg and you are in a coma (asleep), you will feel no pain. You must have a conscious, working brain to feel pain. The brain can also feel things that we know are not there. I am missing one finger but with my eyes closed, my hand "feels" intact. The fact that I can still feel my missing finger does not mean I am crazy. The brain can received signals that cause us to feel sensations and the brain can put out signals that makes us think those sensations are there. We cannot control this. It is well known that some patients who suffer amputation will develop phantom pain. These patients feel pain from a part that is no longer there. This pain is as real as a pain generated by an injured part that is still there.

The illness depression can cause the sensation of pain from any part of the body. Chest and belly pain are the most common examples. Depression can also make pain less tolerable from disorders known to cause pain (e.g., arthritis). Severe, chronic pain can also cause depression which can lead into a vicious cycle of worsening pain. Depressed patients tend to seek medical care for multiple painful or uncomfortable complaints perceived as illness. Rarely do patients seek medical care for emotional feelings that are also clearly abnormal.

Relief from illness cannot be achieved until the correct diagnosis is made. There is no blood test or machine that can confirm depression. Instead, a trial of antidepressant medication is needed. The resumption of normal mood and sleep after antidepressive therapy is the best conclusive evidence that depression was the underlying illness.

The illness "depression" is not simply a mood (i.e. "I feel depressed"). It is an illness of abnormal feelings including, perhaps, feeling excessively "depressed." The tendency for these mood changes to include feeling "depressed" gave this disorder its name. However, usually other abnormal feelings dominate (e.g., anxiety and pain). Feeling really "bad" is by far the most common problem all depressed patients notice.

SWEET TOOTH
BEAUTY PAGEANT

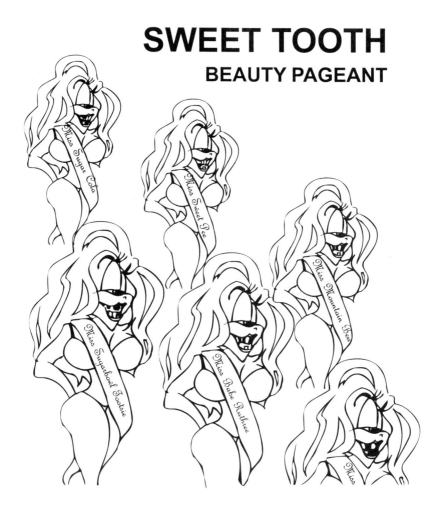

Step 9

66. Beware Depression

Patients who suffer with any long term illness, such as diabetes, are vulnerable to develope depression. Untreated depression is an important, but rarely mentioned, risk factor for heart attacks and strokes (more important than cigarettes). Medical depression, when present, should be treated.

The medical definition of the word "depression" is different than that of the general public. From a medical standpoint, depression is an illness with real symptoms that affects the health of the patient. It affects the rich and poor, the old and not-so-old, blue and white collar workers, and all races. The vulnerability to get clinical depression increases during stressful events. (But not caused by such events.) And a family history of depression is a strong predicator of the risk of developing depression.

Depression is NOT a mood. It is an illness. It can show itself by sleep disturbances, fatigue, excessive worrying about unimportant things, loss of interest in social and pleasurable activities (no motivation), increased irritability, uncontrolled crying, and a decrease in concentration.

Families can have trouble understanding a depressed patient. There is often no sympathy for the depressed person who is irritable and fatigued. Instead, the person is labeled as having a bad attitude or lazy. There are some people with bad attitudes and there are some lazy people. But if those traits were not characteristic of a person before, the family must consider that the person is suffering from depression instead. We know that depression is common. Patients who suffer from depression view themselves as worthless and they want to be left alone. Therefore, they do not seek treatment. They are ashamed to complain about their problems. So depressed patients hide their symptoms from doctor, friend, and family. Doctors miss more than half the cases of depression. It behooves friends and family to be sure a person accused of having a "bad attitude" is checked for depression. Ask your doctor.

Other disorders can alter moods, too. They include anxiety (worry too much), panic attacks (scared to death), obsessive/compulsive behavior (too particular about details), and bipolar affected disorders (manic-depression). All are treatable with medication. None of these disorders should be viewed as "crazy." "Crazy" people — those who walk the roads talking to themselves, etc. — are suffering from something more serious such as schizophrenia. A schizophrenic has trouble communicating socially and he is distracted by hallucinations (imagined demons attacking them or others). They have trouble knowing what is real. They can view themselves as normal when, in fact, they are not. They are out of touch with what is real and what is not.

In contrast, depressed patients realize their moods are inappropriate. They realize they see the cup as half empty when it should be viewed, at least sometimes, as half full. They know there is something wrong. Depressed people do not lose contact with reality. They feel like they are "losing it" but don't. They think badly about the way they feel, but nevertheless, can't control the bad feelings, fatigue and insomnia

In years past, treatment for depression was limited. A famous example of treatment is Sigmund Freud and his psychotherapy which we now associate with "couch" therapy. This treatment is no longer used for depression Then there was the discovery of electricity. Electricity was successfully used as a treatment for depression. Years ago, electric convulsion therapy (ECT) was the only treatment available for depression. Today, it still works in some cases where other treatments fail (which is rare).

The real revolution in the treatment of depression started with the discovery of effective medication. Tricyclic antidepressants (TCAs) and lithium were discovered some 40-50 years ago. These old drugs changed the concept of treating depression from blaming moods to treating it as an illness. In other words, when the chemicals in the brain are adequately corrected, the illness called depression will resolve.

Old medications are effective. Price-wise, they are cheaper. Problems with these medications include annoying side effects (such as a dry mouth, weird dreams, etc.). Excessive amounts can be lethal. But their affordability has merit. For some people, these drugs are wonderful for the successful treatment of depression. There is no shame in using a drug that makes people better.

Newer antidepressants have been developed called selective serotonin reuptake inhibitors (SSRls). They are considered "improved" because there are fewer side effects, and they are safer in the hands of suicidal patients. However, add a "zero" to the cost per month for treatment. These drugs will cost between $70-$140 a month. A famous example of the newer drugs is Prozac. It is a drug that deserves neither its reputation as being the best nor the worst drug (depending on who you listen to). Like all SSRls, it is a good antidepressant medication, effective in 80% of all patients taking the drug.

There are a few other drugs that do not fit into the previous two categories. They are less commonly used, (e.g., trazadone, wellbutrin, buspar, etc.).

A high number of patients will try to treat depression themselves. They will seek and receive sleeping medications, tranquilizers ("nerve medicine"), and/or alcohol. These "remedies" are usually not helpful. In fact, these drugs can make depression worse.

Some people confuse antidepressants with "nerve pills" that are tranquilizers. Tranquilizers give a quick sense of pleasant relief and can be addicting. Some patients build up tolerance to these effects (e.g., it takes more and more of the drugs to obtain the same degree of relief). Patients can also suffer withdrawal from these drugs (if they are on high doses or are long-term users) when these medications are suddenly stopped. Changing a patient, when needed, from tranquilizers to antidepressants takes months, not days.

Antidepressants do not tranquilize. They treat the underlying problem (depression). Antidepressant drugs are safe, rarely build a tolerance in a patient, and do not cause severe withdrawal.

Depression is a common illness that is very disabling. It causes immense suffering for patients and for those people who care about the patient. It is extremely easy to treat with proper medication in the proper dose (e.g., antidepressant).

STEP 9

So what is the proper dose? What is the proper medication?

That's the hard part. We don't know enough to identify which patient needs which medication other than trial and error. It usually takes 3-6 months of "educated guesses" to get the right combination of dose and medicine. A patient must have faith in their doctor (and believe that the diagnosis of depression is correct) to help them through the time it takes to find the best treatment (including eliminating side effects, if they occur).

Without proper treatment, most depressed patients will only get worse over the years. Unfortunately, with time, the brain of an untreated depressed person can become permanently damaged. Therefore, getting proper antidepressant treatment for depression is both very important and very rewarding.

Depression is very treatable, but improvement takes weeks to months (not hours or days). Beware depression! Effective medication is here.

Eat more FISH!

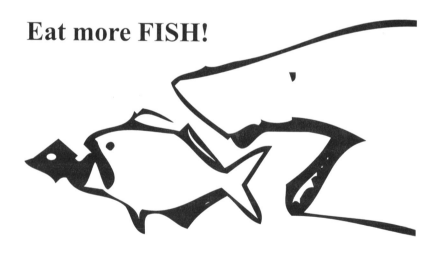

Step 9

If you do not have any pain in life, it is probably because you are dead. All life depends on food. Life can be as wonderful as you are willing to make it. Success depends on *Attitude*. Why we eat affects what we eat. Today is the ninth step towards *your control* over diabetes.

67. Goals for *STEP 9*

Better attitude — read: *13. Fats, Fads, Facts, & Fiction*; *14. The Battle of the Bulge*; *28. If Losing Weight Was So Easy, There Wouldn't Be So Many Fat People*; *15. Why Eat and Drink?*; and *16. Why You Eat Affects What You Eat*.

When human beings become part of the society, they learn from other people all aspects of daily living. Few Americans are Native Americans. Many traditions and diets from other nations disappear when immigrants become "Americanized." Even Native Americans have become "Americanized." American tradition and culture is "As American as Apple Pie." Whatever makes so many people eat like Americans, those forces are very strong (and complex). Americans like to eat. More than half are overweight. Overweight is "normal" in the U.S. Both the number of Americans overweight, and the rate at which this is occurring, are rapidly increasing.

We are what we eat. What we eat, and how much, is not good. Despite America spending more on health care, many nations' (from which we originated) current citizens live longer than we do. At least half of all cancers in America are diet-related. America eats too much sugar, fat and meat. A high protein diet makes forming kidney stones more likely. We eat a lot of meat and pass more kidney stones than any other country in the world. Excessive calories cause obesity. We are #1. Most diets lack fiber (fruit, vegetables, and high fiber bread). This can cause constipation. The U.S. buys more laxatives than the whole world combined (some things aren't coming out right). Whatever the reasons Americans eat (quantity or quality), the harm on health is low on the list.

Step 9

Dieters forget, nutritionally, how badly most Americans eat. Instead, they yearn for traditions "as American as apple pie." Members of any society tend to resist ending lifelong habits (no matter how desperately the change is needed). This hatred for dietary change is what makes diet programs tiptoe around the need for real changes in the way we should eat. For example, the American Diabetic Association (ADA) literature on diet reassures American diabetics by stating "Diabetes doesn't change the kind of foods you eat." That is true, "diabetes doesn't," *but* most American diabetics better "change." What a diabetic should eat goes against a lot of American traditions (including "apple pie"). A good diabetic diet is very different from "normal." Why we eat affects what we eat. A concerned diabetic's primary purpose for eating is to maintain good health. Most Americans choose food for other reasons (e.g., because it tastes good, etc.).

Most diabetics have been eating like "normal" Americans; one reason diabetes is so common. It's not normal for most Americans to eat a healthy diet in moderation (or small meals frequently). A big change in diet can make a diabetic feel like a social outcast. Very strong social pressures e.g., holidays) make healthier diets very hard to maintain. "Diet" can become a four letter word.

Bad attitudes that resist needed change include: I want to eat like everyone else; they should make a diet pill so I can eat any way I want; it is already unfair I have diabetes, "diet" is another form of punishment; I'll just simply die if I don't eat something that only tastes good (good "ol' American crap"); I just want to relax and have fun eating; I hate having to plan before eating; OR I can't do this forever, so I plan to stop dieting once I achieve my goals.

The fundamental mistake most dieters make is that they keep forgetting how badly most Americans eat. Improving attitudes about dieting can help you stay on an *unusually* healthy diet.

Diabetes is treatable (it used to be fatal). The first treatment for diabetes is diet. There is no cure for stupidity. From a health care point of view, it is stupid to eat like a "normal" American. If you eat like a "normal"

Step 9

American, you will probably die like one (only sooner with diabetes). Whose funeral do you want to go to: *yours or theirs*? You need to develop a hatred for how America eats, not how you diet. America has a big need for a new diet, it just hasn't started yet.

The most common problem for good intentions is stupid or bad ideas. If it's too good to be true, it isn't. There are many people who will try to say to you what you want to hear (especially if you are paying for the advice). That will never change what you need to do. Use common sense. A pill cannot fix what someone puts in his or her mouth. If you have a brain, why not use it before you put something in your mouth. Your attitude can choose to either "eat to live" or "live to eat." People who only live to eat don't seem to have much of a life, and it will get even smaller. What we eat affects how we feel. Diabetics can only feel as good as they eat.

Calories always count, whether you like counting calories or not. It is not hard counting calories, you just have to work hard doing it. Life is not fair, some of us must work a lot harder than others to stay alive. Some are much less fortunate, they died young. The correct number of calories needed to control your weight and diabetes is not negotiable. "Trying" doesn't count. You either do count or you don't. In math there is only one right answer. Just because you don't look for calories doesn't mean they are not there. You can't judge food by its cover, you have to look in a book or label to see what's in it. If you can't count calories eating out, don't eat out.

A humorous attitude helps: "The job's not done till the paperwork is done." Keeping a food diary is like going to the bathroom. Are you complaining about *that* paperwork too? NO! The amount of crap you can hold is limited. Crap needs to be eliminated at both ends. You are what you eat when you can't eliminate it (constipated too?). To help solve this problem, do not eat crap (NO crap). What is there about "NO" that you don't understand? The "N" or the "O"?.

The worst dietary mistake for an alcoholic is alcohol. The best treatment is **no** alcohol. The worst thing for a drug addict is drugs. The best treatment is **no** drugs. A common cause of obesity is simply eating because it tastes good. If you are not part of the solution, you are part of the problem. If part of the problem is a "sweet tooth," part of the solution is **no** sweets (**no** plain sugar and **no** artificial sweeteners). Some of the worst food & drink for a diabetic is the "normal" American "crap" full of fat, sugar and meat without enough fiber. Some people are "just dying" to keep eating or drinking this crap (they are much closer to the truth than they realize). The best treatment is **no** crap. Are you dying for food? Smart people eat right. Dumb ones don't.

If staying alive wasn't important, there would be many easy ways to lose weight. If losing weight was easy, there wouldn't be so many fat people. The hardest way to lose weight is to continue to eat/drink like a "normal" fat American. Millions of Americans lose weight every year, only thousands keep it off. There is no such thing as a temporary diet that works. A diet can only work if it is good for you and it is for life. If there is no need to change, why bother? If there is a need, why stop? It takes a lifetime of eating to become overweight, it takes the rest of your life to keep the weight off. Time changes from time to time, fools don't. The safe way to lose weight is to eat only what is good for you and count calories. The best foods taste good and are good for you. Both what and how much counts (Quality & Quantity).

Too much of anything is bad.

Attitude and feelings are not the same. You control attitude, not feelings. Hunger is a feeling that you cannot control. Attitude is "what and why" you eat. When hungry, control "what and why" you eat. Eat high fiber food that is low in calories. This will satisfy hunger regardless of whether it tastes good or not. No one denies it's nice when food "good for you" tastes good as well. But it always matters how much you eat, what you eat, why you eat and when you eat it. Think before you eat. Attitude about "**the diet**" will determine your **success.**

STEP 9

Questions your doctor might ask you:

What are your feelings and attitude?
Are you having any problems with glucose, diet, weight, or exercise?
Do you know all your medication bottles?
Are you finding new things to eat?
Are you eating six times a day?

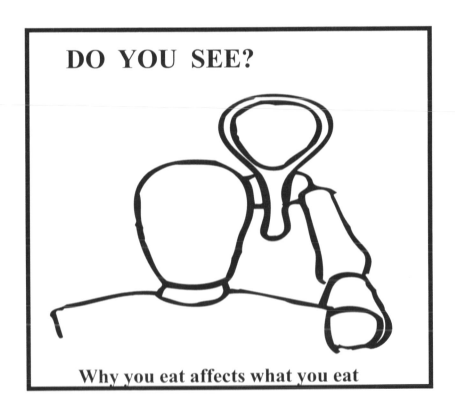

DO YOU SEE?

Why you eat affects what you eat

68. 'Til Death Do Us Part

Ask the average woman what is the leading cause of death for women in the United States and she will probably tell you, "Breast cancer." I asked my (former) wife the same thing and she gave me the same answer.

There are obvious differences between men and women, but the leading cause of death in the U.S. isn't one of them.

Why do so many women think it's breast cancer? I believe one reason is the fear of breast cancer. In years past, treatment for breast cancer was complete removal of the breast (mastectomy) and lymph nodes in the axilla (arm pit). This surgery was deforming and caused long-term problems with the affected arm. Breast cancer is not an uncommon cancer and is particularly lethal when discovered in young women.

The "war on cancer" has mobilized women advocacy groups to focus attention on breast cancer. There is a great deal of publicity encouraging women to have mammograms and perform self-breast exams. This in turn has uncovered numerous breast lumps that require biopsies. Fortunately, only one out of ten lumps is breast cancer.

Detecting breast cancer early is important. Better knowledge of what constitutes effective treatment for breast cancer has greatly improved its treatment. Radical mastectomy (removal of breast and lymph nodes) is now rarely done. Simpler mastectomies or lumpectomies (removing only the lump from the breast) can, many times, provide equally good cure rates and are less deforming alternatives. Chemotherapy is now better than ever. Earlier detection of cancerous lesions is becoming common place, making any treatment much more effective and less deforming.

The fact is that breast cancer, though still a deadly disease, is not as bad as it was in the past.

Today a lot more women smoke than in the past. Because of smoking, lung cancer death has now risen to exceed breast cancer death. ("You've come a long way, baby.") Breast cancer has been relegated to the second most common cancer death in women. The leading **cancer** cause of death in women is now lung cancer. Unfortunately lung cancer treatment and detection have not greatly improved.

The fact remains that cancer has **never** been the leading cause of death for either men or women.

So what is the leading cause of death for women? The same as for men — heart attacks and strokes (cardiovascular disease).

If women want to live longer, they must do more than check their breasts for lumps. Obesity, smoking, and a sedentary lifestyle are becoming increasingly more common. Associated with this are increasing rates of diabetes and hypertension. Therefore, good preventive care requires exercise and good nutrition (not just mammograms).

Unlike men, women can sometimes get a very early warning that they can develop diabetes in later years. Women who develop diabetes during pregnancy are very likely to develop Type 2 diabetes in later years. Maintaining ideal body weight after delivery can greatly reduce or delay the development of Type 2 diabetes.

Heart attacks and strokes kill many more smoking women than lung cancer.

Elevated cholesterol must be more carefully interpreted in women. A woman's total cholesterol on average is normally higher than a man's. One reason is that before menopause, estrogen increases the HDL (good) cholesterol. High levels of HDL cholesterol can offset high levels of LDL (bad) cholesterol. When both HDL and LDL are high, total cholesterol can be very high, yet the risk for a heart attack can still be low.

Since women are not the same as men, lab results have different implications. The predictive value for some cholesterol panel results measured in women is not known (it has only been done in men). Nevertheless, women who do have cholesterol as bad as men can expect to suffer the same consequences as their male counterparts.

It is possible that because estrogen has some kind of impact on cardiovascular disease, women rarely have heart attacks prior to menopause. In any event, heart attacks kill many more men below age forty than they do women. What most people don't realize is that, after menopause, women catch up with men and ultimately share similar rates of heart disease. No one is denying that women live longer than men, but when they do die, they tend to die for the same reasons.

Estrogen seems to play an important role in women's health. Details are still in heated debate.

Earlier studies suggested heart attack risk was reduced by 50% for women who use hormone replacement. Later studies showed women on hormone replacement who were at high risk for heart disease died sooner. I think much work needs to be done...

Another concern about hormone replacement is that it might increase the risk for certain cancers. Increased uterine cancer risk is eliminated with a hysterectomy or with progesterone hormone combined with estrogen replacement. The increased risk for the dreaded breast cancer, if real, is small. Most studies suggest that estrogen does not increase the risk for cancer, but rather, stimulates more rapid growth of cancer, once cancer develops. Faster growing cancers are detected sooner, possibly allowing detection before it has had time to spread. These early cancers have higher cure rates. Breast self-exams and mammograms, for those on hormone replacement, help reduce this concern further.

Hormone replacement will help hot flashes and delay some undesirable changes that occur after menopause. It may slow down some aging, but not without risk in some patients. Hormone replacement might prevent osteoporosis and Alzheimer's. This too, needs clarification.

But all this fuss doesn't matter if everyone is on the wrong boat.

Wise up, women! Mammograms, hormone replacement, breast exams, and PAP smears are not as important in older women as weight control, exercise, cigarettes, cholesterol, diabetes, and hypertension are. Heart disease risk factors are far more important.

Women generally are much better about seeing doctors for preventive care than men are. What's not clear is if women's preventive care is as good as it should be. Is her heart being checked like her breasts are?

STEP *10*

Specialized care has its place in medicine, but the whole picture should never be lost to one part. It is not clear if women who rely on gynecologists for all preventive care are shortchanging medical attention needed for the whole person. In other words, a gynecologist's medical focus on preventing heart attacks may not be as good as a general practitioner's who actually treats these life-ending illnesses (as well as other diseases).

When it's time for a woman to get a comprehensive medical exam (especially after childbearing years), a family practitioner makes a lot of sense. Furthermore, when illness is discovered, it impacts on families, not just patients. It's helpful for women if the doctor is familiar with the whole family. It's also worth noting that a husband is more willing to see the doctor for his illnesses **after** his wife has seen that doctor first.

Common diseases occur commonly. As time passes, this includes the leading cause of death. Ninety percent of all medical problems can be addressed by family practitioners. It's easy to forget the whole when too much attention is given to the parts.

Like it or not, men and women (or husbands and wives) sometimes have a lot more in common than some people think...

'Til death do us part.

Step *10*

69. Confusion about Chest Pain

When a person feels something wrong, such as pain, it is only natural to wonder what the cause is. Because heart attacks are the leading cause of death for both men and women, chest pain is, naturally, of concern. Most people with chest pain, if only for a minute, wonder if a heart attack is a possible cause of their pain.

Harm can be caused when anyone delays the treatment needed for a heart attack. This is especially true today since new treatments for heart attacks are rendered useless if delayed more than three hours. Most heart attacks occur when blood flow to the heart is blocked by blood clots. Drugs can be administered to dissolve the blood clots before irreversible heart damage occurs. However, with sufficient time, heart muscles without oxygen will die. After this point, restoring blood flow to dead heart muscle serves no purpose.

Everyone knows someone who has suffered a heart attack. There are many incidences where delays were made in seeking treatment. Even people having chest pain who are considering the possibility that they are having a heart attack can manage to talk themselves out of seeking immediate treatment. Some of these delays ultimately prove to be fatal. Therefore, chest pain should be of concern to everyone.

Unfortunately, life (and death) is not that simple. Not everyone with chest pains is having a heart attack. Most chest pains are not heart attacks.

Chest pain is not uncommon in children and young adults. Serious heart problems are **un**common in children. Most children with true heart problems have other noticeable problems and do not live with undiagnosed heart disease. Healthy children very rarely have heart problems and heart attacks in these children are extremely uncommon.

A lot of publicity is given to the sudden and unexpected death of a young athlete who had undiagnosed heart disease. The shocking news distorts the fact that these cases are exceptionally rare. For these young people, chest pain is not usually a preceding symptom. So-o-o, chest pain is not a

STEP *10*

risk factor for a sudden heart attack in otherwise healthy young children and athletes.

Chest pain in children deserves to be diagnosed, but "heart attacks" are an unlikely cause.

Many heart attacks do not cause chest pain.

When I was working in the emergency room, I saw one patient who was seeking treatment for his severe diarrhea. In addition, he also had worsening heartburn located just above his belly button. His heartburn had been recently evaluated to make certain that it was not coming from his heart. He had been discharged from the hospital two days before for this; all his heart tests were normal and it was concluded that his pain was coming from his stomach.

The leading cause of law suits against emergency rooms is a missed heart attack. Everyone, including juries, thinks it's hard to miss a heart attack. It is **not**.

This patient had no concern about his heartburn. He simply wanted treatment for his diarrhea. However, as a general rule, any discomfort (including heartburn) above the belly button is a possible symptom of a heart attack. As a precaution, at the last minute, I decided to order an EKG. To my surprise, his EKG was diagnostic for a new and massive heart attack. Unfortunately, even with prompt diagnosis and treatment, this fellow died later that night.

Gee, I wonder how "heartburn" got its name.

Less common symptoms of heart attacks can range from passing out to burping a lot that day. Some people — as far as we know — can have no symptoms at all. Some heart attacks are going to be missed.

Despite all this, chest pain is still the most common (and important) symptom of a heart attack. Heart attacks are common. Therefore, anyone with chest pain is encouraged to seek a doctor. This does **not** mean everyone with chest pain is having a heart attack.

And that's the problem. How do you encourage people to seek treatment without making everyone panic the moment their chest hurts? Let people know what to look for. So-o-o, what are the typical symptoms for a heart attack and who is at risk?

The typical symptoms of a heart attack include: a heaviness, minimal discomfort, or obviously severe pain in the chest; discomfort or pain in the neck, either arm or both arms; excessive sweating; choking or shortness of breath; severe sweating; or unusual heartburn. Generally speaking, these patients feel and look bad.

People at risk — smokers, diabetics, obese patients, age over forty-five (over thirty with other risk factors), men and post menopausal women, sedentary life styles, preceding history of chest pain which occurs with exertion and resolves with rest, family history (at an early age) of heart attack or stroke, elevated LDL cholesterol, low HDL cholesterol, history of high blood pressure, history of stroke, history of previous heart attacks — should be more concerned about any symptoms (e.g., chest pain) of a heart attack.

As with everything else, severity and duration are important factors to consider as well. A onetime brief twinge of chest pain should not be viewed the same as a crushing pain that has lasted ten minutes or more. Accompanying symptoms should be weighed as well, e.g., severe sweating.

Half of all heart attacks are without chest pains. Many chest pains are not heart attacks. Chest pain is the single most common symptom of a heart attack. Decisions about what to do for chest pain are extremely difficult. This also includes the urgency to seek treatment. Do I go to the emergency room, do I call 911, or do I wait to see my doctor?

Chest pain is not synonymous with heart attack and vice versa.

As you can see, there are multiple factors to consider. Possible causes for chest pain fill medical text books. Rule Number One: better safe than sorry. If in doubt, seek medical attention. One possibility for patients who have an established physician is to page your doctor for immediate advice about your particular situation. However, your call cannot always be returned. Therefore, your own judgement may be your only guide.

This article should make it perfectly clear how difficult it is to distinguish many heart attacks from many chest pains. Only hindsight is 100%

accurate. There are no guarantees that anyone can be right about chest pain. This includes when and how to seek treatment and what the diagnosis could be.

But when in doubt, check it out.

You know, it's amazing that I don't get a heart attack just thinking about it.

LIKE FATHER, LIKE SON?

EAT LIKE AN AMERICAN, DIE LIKE AN AMERICAN

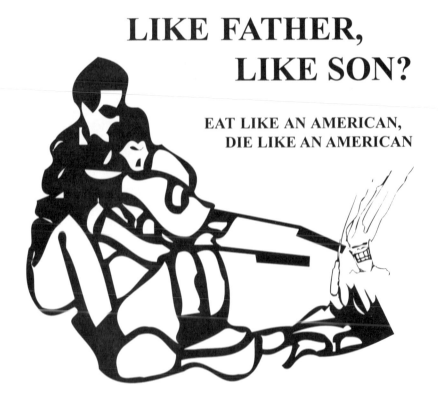

70. Accepting Human Error

Many people think that doctors should not allow mistakes to occur. The more severe the consequences, the less tolerated the error should be. By eliminating error, medical care improves.

Eliminating mistakes is done by many methods. Criminalizing mistakes has become more popular these days. Fines, jail sentences, law suits, demotions, and firings are all good examples of how we deal with mistakes. It is easier to convict people if laws, regulations or policies are written to spell out exactly how things should be done. Stray from one sentence of these documents and punishment can be inflicted.

Psychologists study how and why people behave the way they do. Many interesting experiments have been done to see if punishment can improve performance. Fear can change behavior but there is no evidence that fear eliminates mistakes.

It's always headline news when fatal mistakes occur. These terrible accidents become automatic law suits. Lawyers defending these fatal mistakes advise their clients not to say anything, including "I'm sorry." Failure to follow your insurance company's advice will usually result in loss of coverage. So-o-o, no potential defendant can say "sorry."

Severity of error is difficult to define. Some people would only consider a mistake severe by the consequences it causes. Others would consider the degree of negligence involved. Finally, there are those who would simply let the rules or laws decide what is bad and what punishment should be administered.

The worst mistakes involve death. No one, including I, would be very happy if a loved one died from someone else's mistake or accident. The same would hold true when someone dies from his or her own mistake. In hindsight, these deaths usually seem ridiculously easy to avoid.

Statistics involving large numbers over a large period of time can produce very predictable data. If it happened a million times, it is safe to say it can happen again. Government statistics can roughly predict the

Step *10*

number of people who will die, each year, by accident. In response to these tragic deaths, the government tries to regulate these accidents away. The government does not try to give acceptable human error rates based on past experience. Apparently they believe that perfect safety can be achieved simply by improving regulations.

Recently there has been a series of newspaper articles, in a local daily paper, highlighting accidental deaths in hospitals. The possibility of such deaths is not new. Old movies, such as George C. Scott's *The Hospital*, and malpractice law suits have shared these concerns before.

Now "experts" are analyzing new statistics of some hospitals that are operating under bankruptcy in Philadelphia. The hospitals highlighted are teaching hospitals. I trained in Philadelphia, but not in the hospital featured in these articles. Critics complain that hospital errors are under-reported despite the fact that most hospitals have extensive monitoring systems in place. When errors are documented, they usually are kept hidden from public view. These critics ignore the fact that hospitals' liability insurance carriers would never allow such information to be released without a subpoena.

These monitoring systems, in my opinion, will also produce false reports. There are some hostile employee relationships and some people are successful in making others scapegoats.

Medical mistakes can be fatal. Sick, injured, or elderly patients are a lot easier to kill than healthy, young people. Unconscious patients are very vulnerable to medical errors. Intravenous lines (IV lines) allow minuscule amounts of medication or electrical current to enter the body, bypassing all natural defense systems (e.g., skin, digestive system, etc.). Very small mistakes can result in sudden death.

Incorrectly dispensing medication is cited as the most common fatal error. There are many more medicines to choose from today than in the past. Today's hospitalized patients are much sicker than those in the past. Increased complexities invite increased likelihood of error. There definitely will be mistakes.

Once, a very good friend and physician cited his own error to me when I was a medical student. An insulin order was abbreviated "10U." "U" stands for units. Insulin is always ordered in units so some physicians don't bother writing "units." The "U" was misread by a clerk as an open zero where the word "units" had been assumed to be omitted. The patient received 100 units of insulin, instead of ten, and promptly died from hypoglycemia (insulin overdose). In this case, the patient was comatose from terminal cancer and, unfortunately, his death was very imminent. Nevertheless, this could have happened to an otherwise healthy patient. More than one person was involved in this error. Writing more legibly without abbreviations could have prevented the problem. The clerk should not have interpreted an order poorly written. Furthermore, the nurse administering the insulin and the pharmacy dispensing the insulin should not have accepted this exceptionally high and unusual dose without further explanation.

If a large number of people are involved in dispensing medication, this supposedly helps provide improved safety. Four heads are better than one. It would take four mistakes — not one — to allow an error to occur.

In my opinion, the opposite could offer more safety. One doctor, working with a smaller staff, is much more familiar with the patients. Misreading handwriting is less common. Familiarity with the usual doses of insulin for a known patient makes any sudden change suspicious and more noticeable. A local pharmacy is much more likely to call and question a familiar doctor.

In any event, the fatal error of this patient was documented. This was the doctor's choice since the hospital personnel was unaware of this error (the patient was expected to die). I cannot recall (it's been years) whether he told the family of this mishap. I do know that he warned the entire physician medical staff of the danger of abbreviating "units." He was a competent physician (above average and not error-prone). He wanted to learn from his mistake and share it with others. He never blamed the hospital personnel though I feel that they did contribute to this error. Had this not been a terminally-ill patient, it's doubtful to me that such honesty could have been practical or possible.

Step 10

I realize that some people might feel punishment was in order. I do not. You can't make this doctor any better. The hospital was a well-run institution. Neither would learn more from a law suit. In my opinion, small and large errors with small and large consequences are a normal part of good medical care. If you want **perfect** care, you need to go to another planet where it *may* be available. I can tell you one thing, you will never find it on this planet. I am not always "politically correct" and this opinion can easily be viewed as simply self-serving. But sometimes "forgive and forget" makes more sense than having a measured response to every problem or mistake. This should apply to everyone, not just doctors. Wars would never end without mercy and forgiveness.

Experience is learning from your mistakes. A new doctor, fresh from medical school, has the most current knowledge but the least experience. Old doctors have some outdated knowledge but far more experience. It's a trade-off where no physician is perfect. Even the most experienced physician continues to make mistakes.

How do we prevent mistakes?

The government's solution for eliminating errors is to make everyone write down everything and to have a rule or policy for every possibility that could generate mistakes. I kid you not, one day patients will begin to die because no staff or doctor has time to take care of them. We will **all** be too busy doing the paperwork trying to prevent mistakes. I suppose if patients cannot receive medical care, they can no longer suffer from any mistakes that medical care could cause. But then again, you don't have to seek care...

The plaintiff's lawyers' solution is to bankrupt anyone who has made a mistake. That means everyone. The defendant's lawyer wants to deny that any mistake can exist. Meanwhile, others are looking for scapegoats. No one will find the truth useful.

The truth is that error is a normal part of life as well as of medical care. Mistakes should not automatically prove negligence or incompetence—in physicians or any other workers.

The inability of juries, the government and the medical community to

Step 10

deal with normal human error in a reasonable way is destroying what I call "decent communications."

Decent communications involve truthfulness and the willingness to share (I'm sorry) tragedy, rather than to blame. Blame generates fear. Truth tends to evaporate with fear. The saddest thing to see between people who care about each other is deception. But somewhere, for some reason, we make this happen every day.

He who is without sin, cast the first stone.

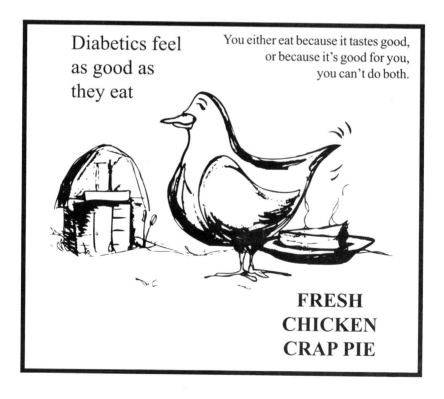

Diabetics feel as good as they eat

You either eat because it tastes good, or because it's good for you, you can't do both.

FRESH CHICKEN CRAP PIE

71. FAILURE TO UNDERSTAND SALT

Everyone knows that water is essential to life. Many people do not realize that salt is essential to life as well. Thanks to mass media "experts," some even believe that salt is "bad." Herein lies the truth.

Living things are constantly absorbing what is needed and eliminating what is not. This is true for every cell in our body as well as for the body itself. Sooner or later water carries everything that the body uses and discards.

Eighty-nine percent of our body weight is water.

Problems begin when our body cannot get what it needs or when the body's capacity to eliminate what it does not need is overwhelmed. Dehydration and "fluid in the lungs" (congestive heart failure) are both well recognized problems associated with water management. When the body has too much or too little fluid, all is not well. The roles of salt and water are intertwined. Every cell in our body controls water flow with salt. In turn, salt is transported and controlled by water.

Soooooo... water controls salt and salt controls water.

The relationship between water and salt is measured in concentration (i.e. the amount of salt that is in water). The inside of every cell must maintain a salt concentration compatible with life (i.e. cell function). Salt concentration outside of an acceptable range leads to certain death. In addition, the total amount of water and salt needs to be adequate. The cell wall protects the needed salt concentration inside the cell from the outside. Our bodies behave in the same way. Many organs (e.g., skin, kidneys, etc.) protect the needed salt concentration inside our bodies from the outside world. If and when we take in too much salt, water, and/or both, our kidney "voids" our mistakes. We urinate.

Salt does much more than control water flow. Salt allows water to conduct electricity. Salt allows cells to generate electrical impulses. The brain and nerves operate by using electrical impulses. Heart contractions and pulse rate are controlled by electrical impulses that can be measured by an EKG machine. Muscles cannot contract and food cannot be absorbed without salt.

As I said before, salt, like water, is essential to life.

Because salt control is intertwined with water control, excessive salt (or vice versa, inadequate salt) can lead to fluid problems and not just salt problems. Depending on circumstances, excessive (or inadequate) salt can lead to abnormal salt concentrations (which can be lethal), excessive fluid buildup or dehydration. Too much or too little water can lead to too much or not enough salt in our bodies. All cells, dead or alive, contain salt. This means that all food (plant and animal) naturally contains salt. There is no such thing as a "no salt" diet. We eat salt every time we eat food. It's a dietary requirement and, therefore, salt is not "bad."

The problem in America is that we add a lot of salt to our food. If there is ever going to be a salt problem in this country, it will not be a lack of salt in our diets. Therefore dietary salt will either be adequate or excessive. Like all good things in life, sooner or later, more is not better.

A well body can be very forgiving toward bad dietary habits. Most Americans have the capacity to eliminate all the extra salt they take in. However, patients suffering from common medical disorders such as heart disease are not so fortunate.

Congestive heart failure (CHF), by definition, is when the heart fails to circulate enough blood to meet bodily needs. CHF will affect kidney function since good kidney function is dependent upon a good blood supply. An impaired kidney cannot eliminate fluid or salt as well as a normal one. Instead, excessive salt can lead to excessive fluid retention — the seeds needed to develop congestive heart failure. Congestive heart failure leads to worsening kidney function which then creates a vicious cycle.

Congestive heart failure becomes noticeable when patients swell or when they become short of breath from "fluid in the lungs." CHF can be life threatening; therefore, patients vulnerable to CHF are very strongly warned to avoid salt intake that exceeds bodily needs.

Both CHF and high blood pressure can be treated with diuretics

Step *10*

("water pills"). The effectiveness of this medication and the tendency to develop side effects are greatly influenced by water and/or salt consumption. Changes in blood pressure and swelling are also noticeable when there are large changes in how much water and/or salt is taken in. Therefore, moderate consumption of both water and salt is wise.

It's logical that people who are vulnerable to fluid problems are therefore vulnerable to salt problems. Once the body's ability to manage salt and water is impaired, greater care needs to be given to what your hands put into your mouth.

The majority of Americans are raised to add an incredibly large amount of salt to their food. For the well, this salt intake by itself is usually not a problem. However, many popular processed foods are now sold that are both high in calories and in salt. The fat, sugar and salt is added by the manufacturer. A good example is potato chips from potatoes. It is the excessive calories that make most processed food harmful to most Americans. However, the excessive salt added is a danger for patients who cannot handle large amounts of salt and water.

Since the majority of Americans are overweight, the quality of processed food is a growing concern. Warnings that encourage people to avoid these products do so for a variety of reasons. The majority of people need to avoid these products because of calories. But calories is a topic much avoided these days. Instead, many people are encouraged to avoid the excessive salt. By doing so, they inadvertently avoid a lot of extra calories. This practice has given salt a worse reputation than it deserves.

Patients taking certain medications (e.g., diuretics) need to be careful about salt. So do patients who have diseases that have weakened organs such as the kidneys. Being careful means avoiding excessive amounts of salt. Whenever dietary mistakes can no longer be automatically "voided" by the body, they must be avoided by the mouth.

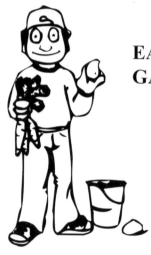

EAT AS CLOSE TO THE GARDEN AS POSSIBLE...

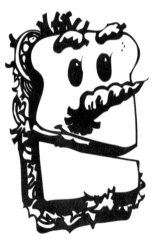

EAT BROWN BREAD...

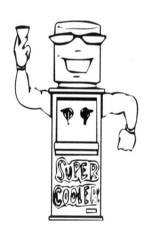

DRINK WATER, PERIOD.

Step 10

72. Time for Thanksgiving

Why do we have fast food? So we can eat and run! Notice how many fast food places there are. A lot of us eat and run.

When nature calls, and you do not have time, you might have a problem.

I have many patients who tell me that they don't have time to go to the bathroom. So what do they do? They "hold it" a little longer. A normal colon lets us know when and where it's time to go. The urge to have a bowel movement becomes weaker the longer it is ignored (and the worse constipation becomes). The bladder is vulnerable to the same problems. An overfilled bladder is at risk of infection. Medical problems associated with constipation (e.g., diverticulitis) and bladder infections are very common. The expense of treating these medical problems is high.

If we live from paycheck to paycheck, we must make more money to meet any extra expenses. More Americans than ever are working longer hours to make extra money. Because we don't have time, we eat out more. This means more fast food and less time to go to the bathroom. To make matters worse, fast food is constipating! Eating out is also more expensive. Therefore, we must make more money to pay for these extra expenses as well. So we work longer hours...

America's "fast pace" for most people is chasing their own tails.

It surprises most Americans that more than half of all millionaires in this country never made more than $30,000 a year. These people were not necessarily "workaholics." They accumulated wealth by not spending it. Some even save money despite generous charitable contributions. These successful people learn to be satisfied with what they have. Being thankful for what you have can save you a great deal of money.

Not being thankful drives us towards getting what we want. This usually means more and/or bigger. In order to pay for this, we must work longer hours...

The Great U.S. Economy that we boast about is sustained by many things that we do not control. One factor we **do** control is "productivity." This important economic factor measures how much each person produces to sustain the economy. American workers' productivity is at an all-time high. This economic per-person figure increases by how many hours we work. The average American worker now works more hours than even the infamous Japanese. If married, it is also increasingly more common that both spouses work. We are so busy working, some of us don't even have time to go to the bathroom. Increased productivity may sound good in the short run but in the long run, it takes a toll on our health. It is doubtful that this kind of increased productivity is sustainable for a lifetime.

It's not "if" we will get sick and die. It's "when." The leading causes of death in America are heart attacks and strokes. Ultimately, there is no cure for these ailments. Eventually they are as fatal as terminal cancer.

The fatal outcome of disease can usually be delayed. Postponing disease itself is by far the most ideal way to stay well. Even though an ounce of prevention is worth a pound of cure, most people claim they do not have time for preventative care. Everyone knows that obesity, smoking, hypertension (high blood pressure) elevated cholesterol and diabetes increase our chances of a heart attack. This really means sooner rather than later.

It's not talked about much, but "stress" increases our chances for a heart attack. Stress is in the eye of the beholder. If we believe something is important, and we have trouble getting it or we are losing it, it's stress. What's important is what we *think* is important. Any failure to appreciate what we have increases our chances of needing more. Ironically, getting more can be at the expense of what we have. It's very easy to take for granted what we already have, for example, our good health. I never appreciated ten fingers until I lost one. Anyone with any ailment will tell you the same.

It will amaze you the things some people wish they had. People with bad lungs appreciate the ability to simply breathe.

Thanksgiving was founded when the Pilgrims learned to survive without famine. Their gratitude was actually directed toward the Native Americans (who ultimately did not survive their good fortune). It was the lack of

Step *10*

food that made the Pilgrims appreciate food. Thanksgiving was **NOT** dedicated to overeating. It was meant to give thanks for what they had (i.e., enough food).

Thanksgiving is a holiday celebrated only in America.

Europe has a high Western standard of living similar to the United States. Europeans eat many foods that are very high in calories and fats (as we do). Traditional European lunch hours differ from ours in that they are two hours long and the meal is the biggest meal of the day.

The life-span of most Americans does not compare well with Europeans. Obesity is not so rampant in Europe. Food and drink before and after lunch is much more modest. Traditional Europeans do not "eat and run" as we do. The risk for heart attacks is much more modest as well.

Obviously, the typical American life style is not a healthy one. By world standards, it's one of the most unhealthy. Smoking, hypertension, diabetes, and the lack of exercise are important problems, but overeating is one of the biggest.

Nevertheless, these other problems cannot be blamed for all of our problems with heart disease. Apparently stress, not seen in other Western countries, plays an important role. The combination of "eat and run" is much worse than eating alone.

Thanksgiving is notorious for eating. But it is also one of the few meals that is relaxed (except for the cook). Many Americans rarely set time aside to *relax* and eat (despite how important stress reduction is). The exception to "eat and run" is the Thanksgiving meal. We just eat. Run is put on hold — **GREAT!**

Now let's put overeating on hold. Take the time to give thanks for what you have.

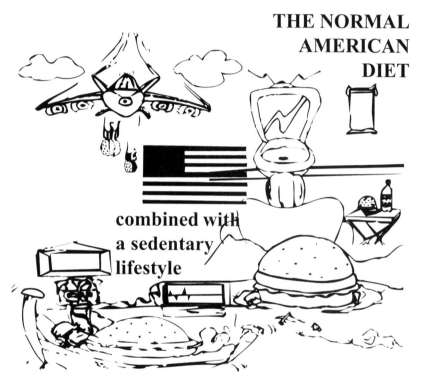

THE NORMAL AMERICAN DIET

combined with a sedentary lifestyle

causes disease and preventable death.

A diabetic feels as good as he/she eats. A good diet is not negotiable. Eat fruit, don't drink it. Eat brown bread. Eat six small meals per day. Count calories because calories count. Always eat as much fiber as possible. Drink water, period. Eat to live rather than live to eat. Remember, eat like an American, die like an American.

73. STEP 10, Finally?

There is plenty of proof that diabetics who kill themselves with a bad diet do not live well. Congratulations! You have completed, but will never finish, Ten Steps for the Control of Diabetes.

Allow me the patience to accept the things that I cannot change.
(I have diabetes.)
Give me the courage to change the things I need to change.
(I need to improve my diet.)
 Show me the wisdom to know the difference.
(see your doctor — review chapters in book.)

Goals for STEP 10:
Review and/or maintain all Ten Steps for the Control of Diabetes.

10 STEPS TO MAINTAIN:

1. Good attitude: Why I eat affects what I eat. I eat to live, not live to eat. I choose to control my diabetes, not let diabetes control my health. Diet is life...

2. Quality food: we are what we eat. Eat a little of a lot rather than a lot of a little (e.g., ADA exchange system). Less (red) meat, more fish, etc. Milk is good as part of a meal. Real eggs in moderation are very nutritious as part of a meal. No juices. No junk food (crap) or sodas.

3. Correct Quantity. Count calories. (e.g., Review carefully counting with a calorie counter and/or ADA exchange system). Your feet cannot outrun your hands.

4. Exercise & increased activity: Forty minute routine for exercise. The same, the same, the same,...(i.e. daily)

5. Preventing Hypoglycemia: eat less, but more often (6 times per day). Regular schedule — energy in, energy out — the same, the same, the

Step 10

same... Don't skip meals.

6. No Crap: if it isn't good for you (it only tastes good), don't eat or drink it. Eat because it's good for your health (nutritious). Less fat, sugar, and meat. Drink water, period.

7. Maintain weight control: diet is for life. The longer you have been overweight, the more strictly you have to maintain a food diary with accurate calorie counts and daily exercise. Eat much less, but more often. Use food scales, measuring cups, and food labels. Eat to live rather than live to eat.

8. Eat more fiber: never pass up the chance. Eat fruit, don't drink it. Eat high fiber cereals and breads. Eat more vegetables. Eat lots more vegetables (count calories)!

9. Periodic home health checks: check feet, check blood glucose, check weight, check calories, and take your medication(s) as directed. Regularly review your handouts.

10. See your doctor(s) as directed: To monitor and refill/adjust medication(s). Check HbA1c, annual eye exam, cholesterol panel, other blood tests, weight, foot problems, blood pressure, other medical problems, etc., and DIET (bring food diary). Your doctor's name and phone number?

Top Ten Most Popular Questions Patients Commonly Asked:

1. Do I really have to change the way I eat? Only if you want to live.

2. What is "crap"????? Food that is not nutritious, and for a diabetic, harmful (e.g., candy, pure sugar..). Food that has had fiber removed and calories added when compared to its "natural" state (e.g., potato chips from potato, juice from fruit ...). Anything high in fat (e.g., fried food instead of boiled, ice cream, pizza ...). Anything high in calories (e.g., pie, "low fat" ice cream, soda, juice...). Colored water — diet soda.

3. I thought juice was good for you? That's what advertisers want

STEP 10

you to believe. Diabetics need fiber. You make juice by removing fiber. Therefore, fruit is better. How many oranges does it take to make one glass of orange juice? LOTS! You would never eat that many oranges at one time. In other words, you would never consume that many calories eating fruit (just drinking it). Reread your chapters from Step 1 (first step towards the control of diabetes) if you do not understand this answer to this question.

4. *Can't you control my glucose with medication (just pills!) without diet and exercise?* As we have said many times, temporarily yes. In the long run, no. Review previous chapters if you don't remember the reasons why. All the building blocks for your body come from food. In the long run, you are what you eat.

5. *Why can't I eat the things I've always liked to eat?* Bad attitude. Quit looking at the things you can't eat. There are plenty of new things you can find that you will enjoy. Use the calorie counter to help you find new things you can eat and like. Review tips in *22. Carefully Counting with a Calorie Counter.*

6. *Can I use sugar substitutes as much as I want?* Artificial sweeteners-sugar substitutes-are not nutritious. Maintaining and satisfying a "sweet tooth" is an invitation for more temptation. A diabetic needs to eat what is good for health, not what simply tastes good. If it tastes good and it is good for you (e.g., fruit) — GREAT! If it tastes good but is not nutritious (i.e. good for you) — FORGET IT. No Crap. Calorie-wise, a diet soda is better than a "regular" soda. But God only knows what other crap is in a diet soda?! There is no evidence that artificial sweeteners/sugar substitutes help people loose weight. If you are thirsty, all you need is water. Water has no calories and it is the only thing really needed when you are thirsty. Again, No crap. Low calorie "desserts" that actually contain fiber are usually okay (such as fruit).

7. *Do I have to do all this "paperwork" counting calories?* Yes, but bad attitude. You cannot continue to improve and maintain your diet without writing it down. Millions of people "diet" to lose weight. Thousands maintain their dietary changes and keep the weight off. Do you complain

about the "paperwork" every time you have a bowel movement? NO! The time spent doing paperwork for either end is important and complaining about it doesn't make it easier. If you stop and think about it, it really isn't that hard to do. Whatever attitude you have about your "bottom" you should keep for your mouth. Both eating and eliminating requires paperwork. You can either laugh about it or cry about it. Laughing is a lot more fun. Remember, only one end should handle "the crap." You choose. Your choice.

8. How can I count calories eating out? Menus and restaurants can sometimes provide caloric information. There is no law against measuring food with food scales and/or measuring cups in a restaurant or at a friend's house. It's legal and moral. Calorie counting must be done (or don't eat out). Many businesses (airlines) and institutions (prisons) can meet your needs.

9. Why do you keep making the diet harder? Because diabetes gets worse, not better. As you get older, unfortunately, there are many things that get worse. Diabetes is just one of those things. Falling apart (with age) won't stop, you can only slow it down. Eventually, your sugar control will become harder to maintain. More medicine will be needed and added. Sooooo.. to keep your diabetes under control, your diet cannot stay the same. It has to keep getting better. Do this before you loose control over your sugar.

10. Why is my sugar so high after hypoglycemia? The body knows hypoglycemia is dangerous. The body has all kinds of ways to try to raise blood sugar when it is too low. Usually, when desperately needed, the body succeeds in raising blood glucose (usually too much). If not, you die. Therefore, hypoglycemia can cause high glucose. High sugar can also cause low sugar. Poorly controlled diabetes can be a "yo-yo" of sugar control (keeps going up and down). This is why diabetics who have poor ("yo-yo") sugar control always feel bad. They also tend to die much younger. Frequent meals with fiber and the right number of calories — on time — is your best protection against hypoglycemia.

STEP *10*

YOU CAN'T MAKE CHICKEN SALAD OUT OF CHICKEN CRAP

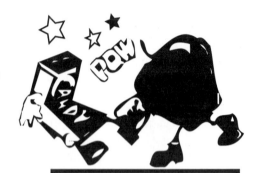

EAT FRUIT, DON'T DRINK IT

DRINK WATER, PERIOD.

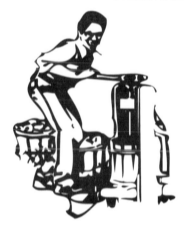

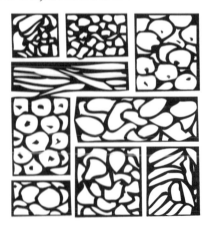

74. CONCLUSION

Think you're done?

Nope. In order to eat to live, it is for life. You are never done. Staying on a diet gets easier, but never easy. There is always something pulling you in the wrong direction. Even your family or friends will do this. The whole country is against you!!!! I don't want to make you paranoid, but they are all out to get you.

So why bother? Because you can't make chicken salad out of chicken crap. You are what you eat.

Read this book. Repetition aids repetition. Reread this book. Look for ideas to keep you out of a dietary "rut." When it is a struggle, it is always easy to get into a "rut."

"Carefully counting with a calorie counter" and "Dieters on a run" are your best chapters to keep you out of a dietary "rut." Remember, if you keep doing the same things you will keep getting the same results. Keep finding new things to eat. A large calorie counter with fiber lists more items you can eat than you can remember. You must find new things you can eat. Then eat it!

By the time you reach the end of this book, you will have forgotten some of the beginning. Rereading a few chapters daily gives you a routine which keeps you vigilant... remember everyone around you might be trying to kill you with bad food.

Always remember that addiction is treated with abstinence. What is there about "NO" you don't understand, the "N" or the "O"?

A good diet is a livelong lifestyle change. Like driving a car, there always seems to be somewhere to go, but eventually you have been there before or you have to go back. The planet is round.

If you would like to give me feedback, write me. I learned a lot more from patients than I learned from the ADA. I will read it, but I probably won't write back. As a physician I have to tell the AMA where I am, so you should be able to get an address from them.

Step 10

If you want to help the ADA, write to them too. They will always write back to at least beg for money....but sooner or later, even "experts" have to learn!

There is no pill that can fix what you put in your mouth, and my book is cheaper.

I want to thank all my patients in Aynor, South Carolina for the opportunity to serve them and all the help they gave me. Conway Hospital, a nonprofit community hospital, made Aynor Family Practice possible. Their dedication to helping this community started this book. I can never forget the great staff at AFP. Judy, Cindy, Pam, Gretchen, Sheila, Ruthie, and Kathy. Thanks to John Eaddy, Wayne Weart, Stanley Tan, and Renee Lamm for professional encouragement. Larry Hardee got me my "wheels." Kathy Dix (Editor, *Aynor Journal*) made my road. John Bauknight helped me drive... I want to thank my neighbors and friends, especially William Hest, Bud and Bonnie Lowe. My family (parents, brother, and sisters) has always been there. Then there is the artwork by Joe Kabriel and Lewis Sierra... My work couldn't leave my computer without the support of someone who actually understands computers, so my sister, Miriam Claude Meijer, Ph.D., deserves special thanks.

Last, but not least, thanks to my wife, Judy Turnbull.

Everyone needs good help, especially me. If you want to succeed in your struggles, find the help you need. At least, die trying...

Recommended reading for physicians:

Davidson, J.K. *Clinical diabetes mellitus; a problem-oriented approach,* 3rd edition. Copyrighted 2000. Thieme.

Can be ordered at www.thieme.com or 1-800-782-3488 (Thieme customer service).

ABOUT THE AUTHOR

Mark Erik Meijer is married to a teacher and has two children. He grew up in Washington, DC and in rural Pennsylvania (his parents immigrated from the Netherlands). In 1984 he earned his Doctor of Medicine from Temple University School of Medicine. Dr. Meijer is Board Certified in Family Medicine. From 1995 to 2002, Dr. Meijer wrote a weekly column on health for the *Aynor Journal* in Aynor, South Carolina. In 2001 he reviewed the results of his diabetic treatment strategies and found exceptionally good results. Now armed with proof of success and a comprehensive diabetes management program, Dr. Meijer is sharing the concepts of his Meijer Diabetes Management Program© with others.

If you would like to write him, he can be reached at:

Mark E. Meijer, M.D.
South Hill Family Medicine
514 West Atlantic Street
South Hill, VA 23970 USA